Nurses and Nursing: Influencing Policy

Edited by

Pippa Gough
Director of Policy
Royal College of Nursing

and

Nicola Walsh
Fellow
Health Services Management Centre
University of Birmingham

Foreword by

Chris Ham
Director
Health Services Management Centre
University of Birmingham

Radcliffe Medical Press

© 2000 Nicola Walsh and Pippa Gough

Radcliffe Medical Press Ltd
18 Marcham Road, Abingdon, Oxon OX14 1AA

British Library Cataloguing in Publication Data

A catalogue record for this book is available from the British Library.

ISBN 1 85775 353 4

Typeset by Acorn Bookwork, Salisbury, Wiltshire
Printed and bound by TJ International Ltd, Padstow, Cornwall

Contents

Foreword

The role and responsibilities of nurses are changing enormously, yet historically nurses have had little input into the way health-care services are designed and planned at a national or local level. This book explores the ways in which nurses can be more involved in shaping the development of health policy. It argues that nurses' knowledge and experiences of patients needs to be articulated and used in policy discussions.

The book is the first in a new series aimed at exploring the dynamic between policy formulation and policy implementation, and the nurses' role within this. This first publication focuses on the development of public health within the current NHS reforms as well as in the European Union. The six contributors identify what knowledge and skills are needed by nurses if their day-to-day experiences are to be used and translated into the central policy-making process. All offer sound and timely analysis as well as some practical ideas on how the nursing voice can be communicated into policy-making arenas at both a national and local level. Themes explored by contributors include: the margin-alisation and visibility of nurses; the need to develop relationships and networks, and to think beyond one's current role; and the need for a solution-focused approach. The editors rightly point out that the challenge for nurses is to shed their victim role and talk not about their problems but the solutions.

The book is unusual as it focuses specifically on policy development from a nursing perspective and will not only be useful to nurses but also to other professionals working in the NHS.

Chris Ham, Professor of Health Policy and Management
Director, Health Services Management Centre
University of Birmingham
July 2000

List of contributors

Sue Antrobus currently works as Co-Director of the Royal College of Nursing's leadership programme and Senior Fellow in policy development with the RCN's policy unit. Before this post she led a team of lecturers/practitioners who were involved in practice development activity. Her current work involves developing nurse activity to influence both policy and practice. She is particularly interested in supporting nurses to integrate nursing practice into organisational strategy and government policy.

Jeni Bremner is Policy Analyst in the Research and Development Directorate at Newcastle City Health NHS Trust. She is currently involved in the development of the Health Action Zone in this area.

Lance Gardner has been a nurse for many years, and has spent the majority of his career working in primary care. He has worked for Kirklees FHSA as a primary care facilitator specialising in developing preventative medicine, particularly in relation to coronary heart disease. In 1991, he moved to Castlefields Health Centre in Runcorn, where he worked for five years as a nurse practitioner. Whilst at Castlefields, Lance became Project Manager for one of the four original Total Purchasing Pilot sites, during which he worked in the practice and the health authority. In 1996, he joined Salford Community Healthcare NHS Trust where he worked as a Project Manager until 1998, when he became part of a nurse-led Primary Care Act Pilot site.

Pippa Gough has worked in a variety of settings as a general nurse, midwife and health visitor both in this country and in

Africa. Her primary clinical experience has been in health visiting, engaged for the most part in public health and community development work. Pippa has also spent a number of years in education as a lecturer in community nursing and health studies. In 1992, she joined the Nursing Development Programme at the King's Fund Centre where she set up the National Nursing Developments Network and acted as external facilitator to a number of centrally funded nursing development units. A year later, Pippa joined the United Kingdom Central Council for Nursing, Midwifery and Health Visiting as Professional Officer for Health Visiting and Community Nursing. In 1996, she joined the Royal College of Nursing as Assistant Director of Nursing Policy, and as from 1 January 1999 she assumed the role of Director of Policy in the RCN's new Policy Unit.

Jane Naish is Policy Adviser at the Royal College of Nursing where she has responsibility for nursing policy and public health. A former health visitor, she also holds postgraduate qualifications in public health and sociology, and is an enthusiastic contributor to the RCN's new MSc in Public Health.

Sandra Rote is a registered nurse, midwife and health visitor. She currently works as a general manager for Northern Birmingham Community Trust. Her recent posts have included Primary Care Development Nurse for a PCG in Birmingham. Sandra worked as a community health adviser for the Royal College of Nursing and was also one of the founder members of the Small Heath Nursing Development Unit, a community-based NDU which strives to integrate theory, research and policy into practice.

Nicola Walsh is a Fellow at the Health Services Management Centre, University of Birmingham. Nicola joined the HSMC in 1996, having previously worked at Berkshire Health Authority and Oxford Regional Health Authority. She has also worked at the Centre of Health Economics and the Social Policy Research Unit at the University of York, where she developed her interest in health policy. In her current post, Nicola is involved in a range of activities – these include co-ordinating and teaching on the health policy masters programme and undertaking consultancy work, working in particular with general practice and PCGs/PCTs. She also leads the national evaluation study of Personal Medical Services pilots.

Susan Williams is European Officer at the Royal College of Nursing. She has been in this post since March 1995. She came to the RCN from local government where she worked as European Officer at the Local Government International Bureau, the European and international arm of the five UK local authority associations. During this time, she developed a particular interest in European social policy.

Acknowledgements

Many people have contributed to the work and ideas on which this book is based, our thanks are due to them all. We also want to thank Sarah Nines and Nandh Rehal for their efficient and enthusiastic support to us both, as we produced this book on top of everything else.

1 Introduction

Pippa Gough and Nicola Walsh

This book is the first in a series that sets out to explore the nursing contribution to health, social and public policy development. We start from a point, synthesised from numerous analyses over time, which sees nursing as marginalised and invisible within the policy process at both an operational and a strategic level in all of our health and healthcare organisations. The outcome of being relegated to the 'wings', rather than being allowed to take our place at the centre stage of health planning and decision making, is that scarce resources are rarely allocated in line with the values held dear by nursing, or in ways which facilitate the delivery of the enormous contribution nurses make to healthcare and health gain.

This chapter starts by briefly examining nurses' current contribution to the policy process and suggests how we can move beyond a policy analysis *of* nursing towards a policy *for* nursing. The rest of the chapter provides the reader with a broad outline of the book and highlights some of the issues to be raised in subsequent chapters.

A policy for nursing

In the past, any analysis of policy and nursing has been confined to a policy analysis *of* nursing, that is centred on a critique of nursing's invisibility and on the way in which mainstream policy impacts on nursing practice and organisation. For example, the 1991 NHS reforms had an enormous impact on nursing under the GP fundholding scheme as the number of practice nurses quadrupled,[1] and the health visitor workforce was cut to the bone. In hospitals, nurse practitioners took over medical roles, whilst the independent sector flourished as we saw the wholesale jettisoning of long-term care from NHS long-stay wards into private nursing homes. All this 'happened' to nursing without nursing or nurses necessarily being instrumental in the central policy-making and political process. What we saw was policy formulated outside of the nursing world and new policies were dropped on to us as passive recipients. The nursing influence arguably only came into 'play' in the implementation of these policies. In the early 1990s, for example, we saw nurses, as ever, mopping up the spillage as the hours worked by junior doctors were cut and nurses absorbed the redundant medical activities. Meanwhile, in general practice, nurses seized the new opportunities presented to them by the 1990 GP Contract. At a local level, many nurses worked hard to interpret and implement policies that improved patient care.

Currently, we see health and public policy formulated within mainstream culture and implemented within our own culture of nursing. Through this process of implementation, policy becomes mediated; we bend it and shape it to fit our own ways of doing and being, which are not necessarily those of the mainstream culture. Figure 1.1 sets out a model to explain this policy process.

The top loop of the figure represents the mediation part of the policy process. Most policy analysis from a nursing perspective examines only this aspect of the cycle. What is explicated more rarely is what happens when we start to feed back into the mainstream policy process our own experiences of implementation. That is, we 'mainstream' our ideas of what works for nursing and what facilitates delivery of our ways of caring; of what enables us to pursue health gain and meet the needs for healthcare. We have suggested that this bottom loop of the cycle is the mediating effect of nursing on

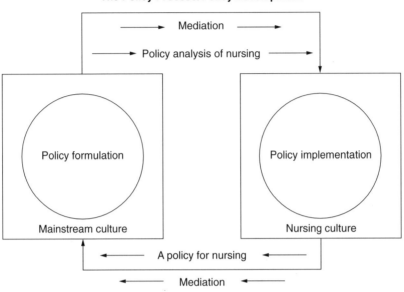

Figure 1.1: Health policy development and its relationship to nursing.

policy formulation. It represents the development of a policy *for* nursing.[2]

If nursing can infiltrate the mainstream culture of policy formulation more effectively, then arguably more congruence between policy formulation and implementation will be the result. If nurses and nursing values are part of the bigger picture, and the political process, then the discontinuity created by trying to implement policy which does not 'fit' with what we do should be minimised. This approach is premised upon inclusion rather than exclusion; on a plurality rather than singularity of views and voices; and on consultation and discussion. In developing this book we have adopted this more inclusive approach.

This book is the first in a new series aimed at exploring dimensions of nursing and its linkage to the political context and thus to mainstream policy. The aim, as stated earlier, is to move on from a policy analysis *of* particular issues relating to nursing practice to develop a policy *for* nursing – thus moving from a policy analysis which merely describes a situation within a particular context, to a process of changing the way nurses interact with the policy environment. This in turn will enable nurses to create more suitable policy frameworks that enhance the contribution they make to healthcare and health gain. This book begins to explore the dynamic between policy formulation and policy implementation and the nurse's role within this.

The book brings together a group of people involved in policy formulation and policy implementation at both a strategic and an operational level. Each of the contributors focuses on a different policy area in relation to the new public health agenda. Although each chapter reflects the individual experiences of the contributors, the group met together and presented papers at a one-day seminar held at the Health Services Management Centre, University of Birmingham, in February 1999. The seminar allowed the contributors to share and debate initial ideas with one another and to an audience of nurses. This sharing of ideas and perspectives enabled a richer analysis to take place and be incorporated into the final draft.

What is presented in the following pages is the start of a process, capturing ideas drawn from current nursing practice. In short, this book represents a policy analysis *for* nursing in an embryonic form which we hope will continue to develop and grow in scope and sophistication over the coming years.

The content of the book

This first book focuses on the development of public health within the current NHS reforms as well as in the European Union (EU). The six contributors have been asked to describe the way in which nursing and nurses can shape the development of public health policy in a way that ensures the nursing contribution is writ large. They were also asked to identify what knowledge and skills are needed by nurses if their day-to-day experiences are to be used and translated into the central policy-making process. All offer sound and timely analysis as well as some practical ideas on how the nursing voice can be heard more loudly within the mainstream public health agenda. As ever, the opportunities are there – we only need to grasp the nettle.

The book begins with an examination by Jane Naish (**Chapter 2**) of some of the past, current and emergent themes within public health and health policy, and their impact on nursing practice. She begins by describing the origins of public health activities as being outside the present framework of biomedicine, concerned as they were with issues such as sanitation and cleanliness 'infused with the twin discourses of eugenicism and preservation of moral order'. This earlier approach within public health was centred on the population, rather than the individual. It had at its cornerstone an understanding of the social and structural context of health, social justice and advocacy, rather than what was to replace it, namely the development of public health science as a medical discipline and the notion of professional intervention to effect 'cure'.

The Thatcherite reforms of the late 1980s created the current public health function. Departments of public health were placed within health authorities under medical directorship. This new specialism of public health medicine pulled public health practice firmly out of the grasp of 'hands-on' practitioners working with communities to maximise health choices. Naish argues that as a result of these changes we saw health visitors and school nurses slowly lose their identity – their community focus. The advent of a primary care-led NHS[3] also contributed to their loss of identity as the redefined primary care was centred on the treatment of illness and management of disease, and so these groups of nurses found expression outside of general practice.

Naish concludes her chapter by looking at the new public health agenda emerging in the late 1990s. This new agenda is characterised by a growing challenge to the dominance of medicine within public health work. Other disciplines and agencies are hammering at the door of public health and questioning the legitimacy of public health as being solely an academic discipline and practice located in medicine. The boundaries of public health are being extended by government policy. It has been openly acknowledged that traditional (medical) departments of public health can no longer meet the new policy agenda alone. Health authorities are to lead the production of a local health improvement plan and work with other organisations to produce such a plan. Nursing approaches to health profiling, community development work and health promotion are all being given a new prominence.

Sue Antrobus (**Chapter 3**) goes on to explore the role of nurses in the commissioning function. She argues that nurses and nursing, far from being the traditional 'gophers' in the provision of services, now have an opportunity to become involved in the commissioning of healthcare services at both an operational and a strategic level. Antrobus suggests that the challenge for nurses is to lift their sights from the operational delivery of care and to use their clinical knowledge to inform and shape the commissioning process. She outlines the nursing action required at each stage of the commissioning cycle: assessment of local health need, the auditing of current service provision, the setting of priorities, development of service and practice, setting of contracts and the evaluation of services. If nurses are involved at each stage of the commissioning process they will, she argues, be contributing to a much broader strategic public health agenda. Antrobus concludes her chapter by suggesting that much work and investment in nurses is needed if this shift from practitioner to nurse strategist is to be achieved.

Sandra Rote (**Chapter 4**) continues to explore the theme of nurses within commissioning by sharing with us her early experiences of being involved in a PCG. She takes us through the commissioning cycle as set out by Sue Antrobus in the previous chapter, but from her unique perspective of personal experience. She demonstrates clearly the conceptual shift needed by nurses to take on a strategic role, which is grounded in everyday experience and knowledge of the health needs of a local community.

In **Chapter 5**, Lance Gardner examines the development of public health nursing from within a Primary Care Act Pilot (PCAP) site. He describes the reality of trying to work using an approach derived from an understanding of the social and structural context of health from within the traditional confines of a general practice. He opens the door on how to influence strategic policy development in line with the demands of his developing practice, and allows us to understand the loneliness and isolation of being professionally 'different'. His work in the Salford nurse-led PCAP truly demonstrates the mediating and powerful effect one nurse and his nursing contribution can have on policy formulation at the centre. At the end of the chapter we are left asking ourselves that if this is the effect of one nurse, what would be the impact of the nursing profession as a whole? As a profession of 650 000 nurses, our collective voice at the policy high table to develop a new public health agenda centred on the needs of the communities we know so well, could be deafening.

Chapter 6, written by Jeni Bremner, broadens our examination of the new public health agenda with a discussion about the contribution of nursing and nurses to the development of Health Action Zones (HAZs). Bremner argues that up until this point there has been little evidence of nurses' involvement in the 'big picture' planning of HAZs. She suggests, however, that their development will offer nurses some new opportunities to push at the boundaries of public health practice and policy, towards the development of a new public service. Bremner draws on her own personal experiences of working within a HAZ area. She goes on to suggest that within a HAZ area, the public health role of the nurse can be used to the full as the focus is on the community and the individual, not just the individual. Bremner concludes the chapter by warning nurses that the path of managed care and doctor substitution is a valid route for some nurses but not for nursing as a whole.

In **Chapter 7**, Susan Williams draws us away from our parochial preoccupations within the UK to consider the development of public health policy within the EU and the way in which the EU has influenced public health policy within the UK. The European Commission's proposed public health framework suggests that the EU concentrates on three core areas of activity in the future, namely:

- improving information for developing public health
- reacting rapidly to health threats
- tackling health determinants through health promotion and disease prevention.

Susan sets out a number of challenges for nurses in mediating the policy process at the European level so that it reflects a nursing perspective. She argues that nursing is not organised sufficiently at a European level to have any lasting influence on mainstream policy. Moreover, there are a variety of conflicting policy networks including a strong and well-established agri-industry lobby which deflects the health lobby time after time. She concludes by suggesting that we have much to learn from developments in the environmental field. The EU has always had much greater powers in the field of environmental protection than have been granted under its public health provisions.

Finally, **Chapter 8** summarises the key themes emerging from these individual narratives.

References

1   Atkin K and Lunt N (1993) *Nurses Count: a national census of practice nurses.* SPRU, University of York.
2   Gough P, Maslia Prothero S and Masterson A (eds) (1993) *Nursing and Social Policy: care in context.* Butterworth-Heinemann, Oxford.
3   NHS Executive (1994) *Developing Purchasing: a primary care-led NHS.* EL(79)94. NHSE, Leeds.

2 The changing role of nurses in public health: past, present and future

Jane Naish

In this chapter I have highlighted themes that have emerged or are emerging in health policy and public health, how such themes have impacted on nursing (or not), and how, in turn, nursing has attempted to assimilate or change them through policy and practice. In doing so I am aware I have been highly selective, and even polemical, in an attempt to illustrate the case for developing a public health policy for nursing. Real life and the everyday context of public health is not, of course, so sharply drawn! The first section of this chapter identifies some themes that have emerged over the course of time to shape the nature, location and function of public health in the UK in the present day.

Themes in UK public health: a brief history

Biomedicine as a model for action and thought defines much current UK public activity. However, the origins of public health in the UK lie outside a biomedical framework of health and disease. Early 19th-century public health activities were primarily concerned with sanitation and cleanliness, infused with the twin discourses of eugenicism and preservation of moral order. Sanitary inspectors/ladies, well documented as the foundation for today's occupation of health visiting, dispensed soap and bibles in equal measure to mothers of the urban poor.[1] However, a focus on the health of a population, rather than merely the health or care needs of an individual, guided their (and others') work, irrespective of the principles and philosophy which underpinned it. This remains true for public health work to this day – a focus on population health rather than the health of an individual (although the meaning of what constitutes the term 'population' is much contested!).

An emphasis on public health as an activity outside the domain and control of biomedicine was confirmed, at least to some degree, up until 1970 when the Local Authority Social Services Act was implemented. Until this time, health visitors, school nurses and medical officers of health were employed by the local authority, not the NHS. Indeed, it wasn't until 1964 when the Council for the Training of Health Visitors issued a new syllabus for the health visiting training course, that entry to health visiting required prior registration as a nurse.

The public health movement around this time was largely made up of individuals whose roots lay within the employment, traditions and culture of local authorities. But over the next decade we saw the birth of organisations such as the Socialist Medical Association, Radical Health Visitors and the Public Health Association, and journals such as *Radical Community Medicine* (now renamed *Critical Public Health*). The chief *raison d'être* of these organisations was, indeed still is, the social and structural context of health, social justice and advocacy, not the development of public health science and professional intervention. This theme, along with the theme of population-based health, has survived to this day, although it is now one of a number of themes in public health and not the overriding or umbrella theme.

Public health as a concern or an activity was not in the mainstream of the NHS until the publication of the Acheson Report in 1988.[2] This report served to refocus public health activities into a professional specialism – moreover, a professional medical specialism. The motives behind this were not necessarily just about extending and consolidating the empire and reach of the medical profession, although certainly that is true. There were also real concerns that public health as an activity remained on the margins of the NHS and lacked power and status within it. The solution devised by the Acheson Report was the creation of a Public Health Department within the NHS, headed up by a medical doctor. The core activity of the new Public Health Department and the new public health specialism was also reoriented towards focusing predominantly on the scientific analysis of population health. It was not intended that this new specialism, public health medicine, would undertake community development work and deliver health promotion messages in any 'hands on' sense with populations. No, the role of public health medicine was to undertake population health analysis (and lead and plan changes arising from such analysis), drawing on the academic/theoretical disciplines of epidemiology, medical statistics and economics (and to a lesser extent health promotion, health policy, and the social context of health and disease).

In the late 1980s, health visitors and school nurses were working within the NHS organisation and not the local authority. Traditionally, these nurses had been regarded as public health nurses. However, with the development of public health departments in district health authorities being located away from 'hands-on' population practice, the perception and belief of health visitors and school nurses as public health nurses was fractured. Public health (medicine) began to move away from an agenda of inclusivity in terms of function and occupational background; the new departments did not include nursing. Another key development over this period was the growth in the specialty of community paediatrics, both the medical discipline and the field of academic research. Measuring (individual) children – in terms of growth and development – became very much the fashion. Health visitors and school nurses all over the country soon became consumed by this new agenda and the (immense) activities it generated. The outcome of these policy developments meant that public health did move into the NHS mainstream, but only in part. Important elements such as advocacy, community-oriented work and non-medical activities were discarded or, in some cases, buried deep within the organisation away from corporate agenda.

The NHS reforms introduced by the Conservative government in 1989 had a huge impact on public health activity. With the introduction of the purchaser/provider split, public health departments located in health authorities were, almost by default, caught up in the commissioning agenda. This, twinned with another emerging agenda, that of effectiveness and evidence-based care, gave public health a new role. This new role involved assessing the health needs and need for care/treatment within a district population, and balancing this against the cost and effectiveness of available health services. All public health departments had to embrace this new agenda, although the extent to which they engaged with enthusiasm for commissioning and effectiveness actually varied across the UK, as illustrated in research by the King's Fund.[3] Interestingly, health visiting and school nursing were the two nursing groups who perhaps came under the closest gaze from the Public Health Department. A number of health authorities, such as Cambridgeshire, 'disinvested in health visiting'; in some instances cuts in services were undoubtedly made reluctantly. But there was also a definite sneer made by some people at this time regarding the contribution of nurses towards health and public health. Even to the extent of posing the question 'what is the effectiveness of health visiting?'. An intriguing but ludicrous question since one can only ask of the effectiveness of interventions undertaken, for example child health screening, and not the effectiveness of an occupational group. The fact that such a question was posed indicates quite clearly the power relationship of (public health) doctors and health visitors. Where else were similar questions posed regarding the effectiveness of public health medicine, surgeons, paediatricians and so on?

The deconstruction of public health medicine?

The 1990s has also been characterised by a growing challenge to the dominance of medicine within public health work. There are a number of explanations for this, not least the drive to reduce health authority management costs through reductions in personnel and skill mix. But, more importantly, challenges have been made against the exclusivity of a unique body of knowledge and skills in public health to medicine. Essentially this challenge has been voiced by public health academics and managers within public health and university departments, frustrated that they undertake equivalent jobs to public health doctors without commensurate levels of pay, status, career structure, progression and development. The challenge has been gaining momentum, aided by the (recent) increased accessibility of Masters degrees in public health – a traditional first training rung for public health doctors – to people who do not hold a medical qualification. Thus, more non-medically qualified people are entering the labour market with higher degrees in public health, who pose an attractive option for employment simply because they can be paid less than doctors – the threat to public health medicine consequently increases. Indeed, such has been the momentum that there is now an organisation called the Multi-Disciplinary Public Health Forum, specifically set up to lobby for commensurability between public health doctors and other public health department employees (*see* Klim McPherson and John Fox for further discussion[4]). This new organisation is already having an impact, for example the Faculty of Public Health Medicine has decided to allow public health professionals who do not hold a medical qualification to sit its exams and become associate (not full) Faculty members, a necessary step at present for career progression within public health departments. The Department of Health has commissioned a study to investigate the measurement of competency in public health personnel who are not doctors; and the Department of Health strategy group, led by the Chief Medical Officer to consider the function of public health in England, now has membership wider than public health medicine. However, it is important to note that, powerful and articulate though this challenge to medicine may be, it is not essentially a challenge to the location of public health or its scientific focus. This challenge therefore poses a dilemma for nursing, which is returned to later.

Other challenges to public health medicine have also emerged, although more diffuse in nature. One of these challenges could be described as the deprofessionalisation of public health, in that it aims to bring the voice(s) of the public into public health matters. This has always been at the core of community development initiatives in health, but has been revitalised by, for example, suggestions from the King's Fund and other organisations that the creation of 'citizens' juries' would enable the public to debate and have a say in local health matters and issues. Certainly media coverage of health-related issues has never been greater and at least some sections of the public can be very well informed and vocal on health issues, if they choose to do so (visit the Internet before you visit your doctor?). An effect of this is to move knowledge, and thus power, away from doctors and other healthcare professionals into the public domain, and as a consequence weaken claims to a unique and exclusive body of public health expertise.

A further diffuse, indeed subtle, challenge to public health medicine comes in the guise of the Labour government. For the first time we have a Minister for Public Health who is charged with taking forward health improvement strategies which require cross-agency working. We also now have a government that recognises – at least to some degree – the social context to public health. Inequalities in health are back on the health policy agenda and a good example of this is the introduction of initiatives such as HAZs and the Surestart Programme, both targeted at vulnerable and economically deprived communities. This is public health in a wider, more rounded sense than at any point in the past 20 years, and it is certainly not the sole province of public health science and analysis, service commissioning or an agenda of clinical effectiveness. The boundaries of public health are being extended by government policy, and it is questionable how public health medicine and traditional public health department functions will fit within them. They are certainly unlikely to remain the only players centre stage.

Public health consciousness in nursing policy and practice

Public health has been a feature of thinking within nursing as far back as the writings of Florence Nightingale.[5] Its overt articulation has not, however, been consistent in nursing policy and practice. We have already mentioned the emergence of health visiting in the NHS and its involvement in campaigns to highlight the political, economic and social context of public health (*see* Drennan for a further discussion of this[6]). We now look more carefully at nursing developments related to the articulation of public health since the 1980s.

This process really began with the publication of *Whither Health Visiting?* by Shirley Goodwin in the journal of the Health Visitors Association.[7] The article was groundbreaking for its time, in that it challenged health visitors to go back to their roots in public health. Goodwin asserted that the health visiting profession had become drawn into routinised and task-orientated maternal and child health nursing which bore little relationship to population health needs. The article provoked passionate and wide debate among health visitors (partly because its author, Shirley Goodwin, was the charismatic and well-respected then General Secretary of the Health Visitors Association). Publication of literature on health profiling as a method of reclaiming public health as the central core of health visiting soon followed this article.[8] Essentially, health profiling was an attempt to gather information on the health needs and views of a small population; plan and prioritise appropriate interventions; and evaluate them. Similar in some respects to the function of public health departments, it differed somewhat in that it had a more local, practice-based and client-centred context, which attempted to incorporate the views and wishes of a local population. The person undertaking the assessment – the health visitor – was also the person undertaking the practice. In other words, it did not attempt to divorce public health analysis from public health practice.

Health profiling was enthusiastically embraced by many health visitors and was influential in bringing public health conscious-ness back into health visiting policy and practice. However, in some senses it failed to meet such expectations, not because of lack of enthusiasm and fervour, but because it did not fit into any supportive structure within the NHS organisation. For the most part, health profiling relied on the efforts of individual health visitors, working in isolation outside of a corporate or conceptual framework of public health practice. Health profiling did not bring together the work of health visitors and public health departments, and health profiles were often disparaged rather than encouraged by the latter on the grounds of epidemiological validity and scientific rigour. However, health profiling did begin to challenge the notion that health visitors and their public health work meant following the plans, decisions and instructions of public health departments and NHS managers: the seeds of public health as an activity which spanned health policy and nursing practice were sown.

It was the birth of the concept of the Nursing Development Unit (NDU) which was to further revitalise the public health function and contribution of nursing. Specifically, the birth of the first three community NDUs in Strelley, Small Heath and Stepney. Each was funded and supported by the King's Fund to develop a vision and strategy to span policy and practice to meet the health needs of their locality. Each used health profiling to assess the local health needs. But perhaps more importantly, each of the NDUs developed the notion of teamworking; they also involved the local communities by translating information on population health into practice. All three units developed a shared vision of public health, which spanned public health analysis and practice, although this was articulated and implemented differently in each community NDU. For example, in the NDU in Strelley, a public health nursing post was developed. The remit for this post-holder was to develop public health information, intelligence and analysis; to support and train local people such as GPs, local authority workers and shopkeepers; and to influence local policies and politics which impacted on health.[9] For Stepney and Small Heath, this was a function and activity of the whole team, not a specific post. The community NDUs were held up as a beacon for how community nursing should, and could, be developed in the future. However, there was no national framework or steer to take these developments forward, so those who tried to emulate the work of the three community NDUs found themselves on the margins of mainstream NHS work (as did the three NDUs within their own trusts – the agenda moved on). This type of community nursing work – spanning the collection of information, policy analysis, community involvement, practice, reflection and teamwork – continues to operate at the margins of the NHS today. It is still, however, characterised by short-term, project-type funding, plus enormous commitment on the part of the individuals involved.

The three community NDUs have had enormous influence on the articulation of nursing policy and practice, and public health. Each had been involved with, and supported by, the Royal College of Nursing (RCN) and as a consequence, in 1994, the RCN set up a Public Health Interest Group to bring like-minded nurses together to network and share ideas on policy and practice in public health. It started a newsletter to encourage networking and information exchange (to this day the only regular publication explicitly on nursing and public health), and published a policy statement on nursing and public health[10] which was a landmark in attempting to articulate policy and practice, and nursing in public health. This RCN publication was not an attempt to create a new specialism of public health nursing, but an attempt to articulate policy and practice across the spectrum of nursing and the spectrum of public health. It identified three separate, non-hierarchical strands and points of engagement within public health and within nursing. The first was that public health concepts and knowledge should underpin all nursing interventions, regardless of whether the nurse is explicitly engaged, or recognises herself as involved, in public health. The second was that community nursing could span the analytical function of the public health department and public health practice at a local, community-based level. The third and final strand was about how nursing could engage in the analytical and scientific work of public health departments, alongside other professional disciplines. The publication also recognised that not all of these strands were exclusive to nursing but that nursing did have an important role.

Following the RCN publication, the Department of Health also published a document on nursing and public health[11] supporting many of the themes highlighted in the RCN publication. This was an important landmark in policy terms since the publication of the Department's document served as a formal recognition and legitimisation of a relationship between nursing and public health (whatever that relationship may be).

Since that time, the development of a policy and practice relationship between nursing and public health has continued, albeit in a largely unco-ordinated and invisible manner. For example, the Department of Health has held several seminars and strategy meetings on 'the way forward'. Some nursing posts specifically designated as 'public health' have been created, both in health authorities and community trusts. The English National Board for Nursing, Midwifery and Health Visiting has also commenced a research project investigating the public health content of health visitor, practice nurse and district nurse education. The RCN has designed a Masters degree programme in public health for nurses and this started in September 1999. All of the NHS regions in England have been asked by the Department of Health to conduct an assessment of where they are with nursing and public health. Nurses are now much more aware of public health issues and much more confident in articulating their contribution – at a national level nurses are represented on most, if not all, major committees and groups concerned with public health, which would have been unthinkable 15 years ago. A relationship between nursing and public health is beginning to emerge. The question is, what do we want from that relationship and where do we go from here?

Back to the future: contradictions and opportunities

There are both opportunities and contradictions in the development of a policy for nursing and public health in the future.

Below, I have set out what I think the opportunities and contra-dictions ahead are; it is for you, the reader, to debate and take these forward.

First, the opportunities. These stem from the shift in govern-ment thinking on the organisation and delivery of healthcare to take on board the social context of health. The creation of HAZs, the introduction of Surestart and the development of primary care trusts (PCTs) are all policy initiatives that present major opportunities for nursing to develop public health leader-ship in policy and practice. This is because they allow, if not promote, a community development approach which mirrors the core values espoused within nursing of collectivism and empowerment. They do not separate structures for policy and analysis from practice (see later chapters by Sue Antrobus, Sandra Rote and Jeni Bremner). This new developing model of public service delivery holds many opportunities for nursing to develop leadership in the future.

What are the contradictions? One contradiction relates to the dangers inherent in claiming a unique, exclusive or specialist role or career pathway for nursing and public health. At a time when the boundaries of what constitutes proper public health work are extending, the multidisciplinary and inclusive nature of public health is emphasised and the dominance of public health medicine challenged, it would be ironic and rather ludi-crous if nursing suddenly stepped forward to claim *it* owned an exclusive body of knowledge and skills in public health. Nursing can span the practice/policy as well as the professional/lay divide in public health – it does not have to enter an either/or argument about the nature of public health as an epidemiolo-gical science versus community development. Personally, there-fore, I am wary of nursing throwing in its lot with the Multi-Disciplinary Public Health Forum mentioned earlier, which does not essentially challenge the traditional focus of public health departments. But how then does nursing develop a frame-work to nurture nursing leadership in public health without tying itself into specific structures? There is another inherent contradiction here in that if nursing and public health is, in one sense, everywhere without any particular distinguishing marks, it can remain nowhere, so to speak, in terms of leadership, and thus remains invisible. To make ourselves *visible* in public health might mean we need to develop career pathways; the creation of posts such as Directors of Public Health Nursing is a possibility. Such a post would (it is hoped) encourage the development of a research base, and attract nurses to specialise in public health. Visibility may come from educational programmes – within and outside of nursing – since formal education might lend some credibility, if only in terms of speaking the (accepted) language of public health, that of case –control studies, confidence intervals and so on. But this then begs the question of education to do what? It defeats a holistic and community-centred approach which takes on board policy *and* practice in nursing *and* public health (and science *and* community development). Perhaps the solution is multifaceted. I do not have 'the' answer. However, it is clear that our aim should be to secure a future for nursing in leading a public health agenda which can reflect our nursing values and what matters to the patients, clients and communities with whom we work. The notion that public health policy is something which nursing merely carries out without influence or involvement should be laid firmly to rest.

References

1 Clark J (1973) *A Family Visitor*. Royal College of Nursing, London.
2 Committee of Enquiry into the Future of the Public Health Function (1988) *Public Health in England*. DHSS, London.
3 Levenson R (1997) *Developing Public Health in the NHS: the multi-disciplinary function*. King's Fund, London.

4 McPherson K and Fox J (1997) Public health: an organised multi-disciplinary effort. In: G Scally (ed) *Progress in Public Health*. The Royal Society of Medicine Press, London.

5 Nightingale F (1893) Sick-nursing and health nursing: a paper read at the Chicago Exhibition, 1893. In: L Ridgley Seymer (ed) (1954) *Selected Writings of Florence Nightingale*. Macmillan, New York.

6 Drennan V (1988) *Health Visitors and Groups: politics and practice*. Heinemann Nursing, London.

7 Goodwin S (1988) Whither health visiting? *Health Visitor*. **61** (December).

8 Twinn S, Dauncey J and Carnell J (1990) *The Process of Health Profiling*. Health Visitors Association, London.

9 Boyd M, Brummel K, Billingham K *et al.* (1993) *The Public Health Post at Strelley: an interim report*. Nottingham Community Health Trust, Nottingham.

10 Royal College of Nursing (1994) *Public Health: nursing rises to the challenge*. RCN, London.

11 Standing Nursing and Midwifery Advisory Committee (1995) *Making It Happen: the contribution, role and development of nurses, midwives and health visitors*. Department of Health, London.

Further reading

Acheson D (1998) *Independent Inquiry into Inequalities in Health Report*. The Stationery Office, London.

3 Commissioning healthcare services: nurses as strategists, operating between policy and practice

Sue Antrobus

Commissioning has become a legitimate part of the *New NHS* language following the Labour government's proposals to introduce local commissioning schemes throughout the UK.[1–4] Yet, although the language is being used, it is argued here that the complexities of the commissioning process, together with the impact that effective commissioning will have on clinical practice, are all factors that are poorly understood by the majority of clinicians and managers operating in the NHS today.

This chapter seeks to examine the implementation of commissioning as a key policy initiative from the perspective of a particular clinical and managerial group – nurses. It is proposed that nurses, in both operational and strategic roles, are vital to ensuring commissioning policy actually happens in practice. This has become even more important with a policy shift towards greater devolution and more locally sensitive commissioning. In setting out the case for the involvement of all nurses in the commissioning of healthcare services, the particular challenges facing this professional group as they do so will be identified and explored.

The importance of commissioning

Commissioning is a strategic activity that frames the whole process of service development within the NHS – or it should do. It is a term that has been confused with purchasing and yet the two activities, commissioning and purchasing, are distinct. Commissioning is a long-term solution. It is a cyclical process involving a whole range of activities. The starting point is the assessment of the health and healthcare needs of a defined population and the end point is the evaluation of the services developed in response to that assessment. Box 3.1 outlines each stage of the commissioning process.

Box 3.1:   The commissioning process

Step 1   Assessment of health need
Use evaluated health needs assessment tools to assess the needs of the population the PCG covers. Collate and review the information obtained.

Step 2   Auditing current service provision
To obtain a picture of what is currently provided, audit service provision collaboratively with other key stakeholders. Map the results of this with the results of the health needs assessment from Step 1.

Step 3   Setting priorities
Not all services identified by the process of health needs assessment will be commissioned. Different priorities will be identified dependent on national and local health need. It is important that the priority-setting process is transparent and the values and principles, which guide decision making, are made clear.

Step 4   Service and practice development
Once priorities have been identified, the next step is service development and within this, at a more macro level, practice development.
This will involve the production of a strategic plan developed by all
stakeholders, both those involved in service delivery and those using
the service. Within the plans for service development will also be
plans for practice development based on evidence of clinical effectiveness in relation to the service being developed.

Step 5   Contracting process
At this stage the services planned are agreed with providers, in the
form of a contract. Providers should have been involved with the
whole process of commissioning so far. The involvement of providers in the designing of services from the outset means that the
contract becomes the vehicle for planned change, jointly agreed
and negotiated between providers and commissioners.

Step 6   Evaluation of the services
The last stage is evaluating the service that has been developed.
Auditing those services and mapping against identified health need
completes the commissioning cycle.

The strategic activity of commissioning is long term, involving
the planning and realigning of services in order to meet both
the health and healthcare needs identified by local people and
national priorities. Purchasing, however, set within the context
of commissioning, is an operational activity. It involves using
existing resources to buy services that are currently provided. It
is a vital activity therefore in the contracting and buying of pre-
existing services, but is not a term that adequately reflects the
activities involved in the development of new services. This
clarity of definition is important to grasp because it is the shift
from purchasing to commissioning at a local level which will
have major implications for nursing practice.[5]
    The commissioning of healthcare services will be one of the
main tools used by the Labour government to address health
inequalities and maximise value for money. In contrast to the

purchaser/provider split introduced by the Conservative government in 1991, the commissioning of services will be done in partnership with other agencies. It is imperative therefore that the commissioning function of a health authority or a PCG/PCT is strong and effective.[6] But what makes for strong and effective commissioning organisations and what to date has been nurses' involvement in those organisations?

The involvement of nurses in commissioning

In the UK, there is no statutory requirement for nurses to hold a board position in health authorities or health boards. This has led to a situation where only about a third of health authorities, or their equivalent, across the UK have a nurse operating in an executive position.[7] It is worth examining the reasons why this might be, before considering the position of nurses within the current local commissioning structures.

One of the main reasons that nurses do not have a seat on the executive board within health authorities, it is argued here, is due to a lack of understanding of the commissioning/nursing practice interface by policy makers, health service managers and nurses. Commissioning, as stated earlier, is a strategic activity, yet a closer analysis of the commissioning cycle reveals that to effectively commission for a population will not only depend on accurately identifying the health needs of that population but also developing and providing that service at a more micro level – to the individual patient. It is clear then that commissioning decisions taken at one level will influence the operational work of clinicians at another level. The position of clinical nurses within this is clear. Nurses deliver the majority of patient care and therefore as a group exert considerable influence over whether commissioning targets will be met within clinical practice. That is, at an operational level, nurses are essential to the success of the commissioning process.

If nurses are vital to commissioning at an operational level then, it is argued here, they are also vital to commissioning at a strategic level – within health authorities and health boards as well as in the more local commissioning groups. It is imperative that nurses are part of the management board of health authorities and local commissioning structures, as it is they who can translate the impact that strategic commissioning decisions can have on the lives of local people and, as importantly, the clinical impact of such decisions. To do so successfully, however, requires nurses to be strategic thinkers. Nurses need to have a broad knowledge and understanding of public health so that they are able to think in terms of the health and healthcare needs of the population rather than the individual. They must also have the ability to interpret and translate the knowledge they hold about the health needs of the population and the care requirements of individuals to health service managers and other clinicians.

If nurses at an operational level are led strategically by a nurse on the commissioning board, their contributions will be able to be moulded in a direction that ensures that the health improvement targets set by the commissioning body are met. Information about the needs of local communities and the impact of policy decisions will need to be well communicated by both groups of nurses (the strategists and the operationalists). The 'cash and care' consequence of commissioning organisations not achieving health improvement targets in practice seems too great to forego the strategic contribution that nurses can make.

Goodwin[8] has proposed a second reason why nurses do not have an executive statutory position in health authorities. She states that there are two groups of nurses in commissioning – the generalists and the specialists. The generalists have pursued general management careers. On the whole, she argues, they think more strategically about how services are organised, their nursing background bringing added value to this work. The specialists, on the other hand, work at an operational level and use their specialist knowledge as an important source of expertise for contracting and specifying and monitoring clinical standards.

Interestingly, the Griffiths reforms[9] reinforced the confinement of nurses to operational specialist roles. The capacity of nursing to influence the future NHS was severely limited at this point as nursing management was swept away.[10] A broad account of the impact the Griffiths reforms had on nursing and medicine found that the impact on each professional group was characterised in many ways by the different styles of nurses and doctors. Doctors were confident and assertive with a history of handling managers and making demands. In contrast, nurses were unconfident, hesitant and deferential, hiding behind hierarchy and unable to turn their numbers and budgetary importance to any distinct policy advantage.[11]

The confinement of nurses to operational roles and functions, together with their lack of leadership skills, has limited the pool of nurses with the expertise and experience to contribute to strategic thinking – a key competency required for commissioning healthcare. It may be that there are not enough nurses with the skills required to commission healthcare. Nurses may also be far more comfortable working in operational roles that are closer to the patient.

Goodwin[8] believes that the operational confinement of nurses is compounded further by the fact that nurses have great difficulty in articulating what they bring to healthcare decision making and policy making. This often means that the contribution nurses make is not recognised by other influential parties. Defining the expertise nurses have and are able to bring to policy and strategic decisions is necessary in order to justify their representation, yet it is something that nurses have been reluctant or perhaps unable to do.[5]

There are several challenges facing nurses then as the new

commissioning agenda takes hold. The first challenge is concerned with demonstrating a much broader political awareness. Nurses will need to understand the direction of public policy in relation to public health and the mechanisms proposed at a policy level for improving health through the structural and cultural changes taking place within the NHS. Within the context of commissioning, this means understanding both the commissioning process and the complexities of commissioning, and then translating the impact commissioning decisions will have on nursing practice at the point of delivery.

Once an understanding of commissioning has been acquired and the impact of commissioning decisions understood at the level of nursing practice, the next challenge is to identify the leadership skills necessary to operate effectively in a commissioning role. It is apparent from the previous analysis that one of the skills nurses require is the ability to operate with a broad strategic focus. Nurses traditionally have the ability to operate successfully at an operational level, for this level defines the clinical work they do. Thinking strategically, however, will enable nurses to use their clinical knowledge to actively contribute to population health gain. This will enable nurses as strategists to feed their clinical knowledge about the health needs of individuals into a population-focused commissioning framework.

The third challenge for nurses is one of language. Finding a language which expresses concerns of a caring nature within a commissioning dialogue, where business expertise is valued, is a challenge for nurses, but one that needs to be overcome so that nurses can demonstrate their particular contribution to population health gain. This challenge is complicated further by the priority-setting process involved in commissioning decisions. Nurses will be contributing to decisions about where resources are allocated. Nurses have not been prepared for this, either educationally or emotionally.

Indeed, the education of nurses emphasises the importance of meeting the health and healthcare needs of each individual patient they care for. This is the same for all healthcare professionals, including doctors. Prioritising services based solely on need will mean that nurses and other clinicians are actively involved in decisions about striking a balance between the quality and cost of care. It will also mean directing resources in response to local need in a cost-effective manner. Doing so, however, may involve reducing the quality and/or cutting the range of services provided. Setting priorities may therefore not sit comfortably with the values of nursing and perhaps is one of the major challenges to nurses' involvement in commissioning roles.

A further challenge facing nurses is to overcome aspects of their socialisation. As a neophyte profession, nurses have been developing their credibility as a professional group. Pursuing professional status has caused tensions to develop between nursing as a profession and the needs of the population. This has been acted out in many health authorities across the country. The tension between nursing and commissioning priorities has led many health authority chief executives to dismiss nurses as they have been unable to operate in strategic commissioning roles where decisions concerning health gain, not the needs of a professional group, are paramount. Nurses, it seems, find it difficult to move beyond their desires to advance nursing when the commissioning debate is concerned with improving the health of the population, potentially at the expense of nurses and nursing. Box 3.2 summarises the challenges facing nurses as they enter the commissioning arena.

The challenges outlined in Box 3.2 are by no means exhaustive, but are some of the topics highlighted in research about the role of nurses in commissioning.

Commissioning in the *New NHS*

It is against this background that the Labour government is inviting nurses to become involved in the development of local

Box 3.2:   The challenges facing nurses in commissioning

- Political naivety
- Operational
- Individual
- Professional focus
- Language of care
- Disease orientated

- Political sophistication
- Strategic
- Population
- Health gain focus
- Care and corporate language integrated
- Public health orientated

commissioning schemes. Although this discussion is focusing on the arrangements in England, it should be noted that commissioning arrangements in Wales, Scotland and Northern Ireland are all different – and the nurses' role within them differs.

In England, nurses have up to two seats on the board of a PCG. The three key functions of a PCG are:

- to improve the health of the local population
- to commission healthcare services
- to develop primary and community care.

In April 1999, PCGs replaced the GP fundholding scheme. PCGs involve groups of practices working together, covering a geographically defined area. They are to build on the successes of fundholding, locality commissioning, and total purchasing projects and other local commissioning schemes. In contrast to earlier local commissioning schemes, PCGs are to involve nurses. Community nurses are to work in partnership with GPs, social service managers, health service managers and lay representatives. As part of the PCG board, nurses will be helping to shape local services in a strategic capacity.

In the *New NHS*, health authorities that have traditionally been the commissioning bodies are to work differently. They are to devolve their commissioning powers to PCGs/PCTs and involve them in the production of the local Health Improvement Programme (HImP). The HImP should provide a direction of travel for the PCGs/PCTs and a framework in which they must work. Those involved in the delivery of care, particularly nurses, should help to mould the HImP so that it reflects the perspectives of the local community and the experiences of service users. A PCG/PCT will also have its own plan, the primary care investment plan; again this should reflect the healthcare needs of the local population as well as the views of healthcare professionals and service users.

The role that health authorities adopt in these new arrangements will have an impact on the ability of the PCG/PCT to commission healthcare services. On the one hand, health authorities are being encouraged to be facilitative and to devolve as much of the commissioning as possible to the PCG/PCT. Yet, health authorities also have to monitor the performance and expenditure of PCGs/PCTs. Health authorities are therefore treading a fine line as they try to operate in both a facilitative and a monitoring capacity.

It is apparent that health authorities will become leaner. They will also become more clinically orientated and public health-focused in their work. The strategic framework within the health authority – the HImP – will need to be developed by a 'bottom-up' process. Such an approach to strategy development is quite different from the way in which health authorities have outlined their strategic direction to date. Health authorities have on the whole operated a 'top-down' approach to strategic planning. That is, they have outlined a direction from the dictates of national priorities and local population data. This approach has been detrimental to meeting the local healthcare needs of the local population. A 'top-led' approach did not engage with the realities of the lives of local people.

A district nurse illustrated to me the way in which she believed PCGs would be far more effective at actually meeting local priorities. Using cervical cancer as an example of a health priority, she described the service development plan produced by the health authority. It had been formulated around a cervical screening programme based at the local hospital. From her experience of working with women locally, she knew that this plan for service development, although logical, would not work in practice. The lay health belief, which these women held, was that cervical cancer was like a lottery and in their eyes a screening programme would make no difference to their health. A further complication was that the deprivation of the particular group the health authority wanted to target was such that these women did not even have the bus fare to make the journey to the hospital, even if they believed the screening programme was effective.

This district nurse believed that undertaking a health needs assessment through the PCG/PCT at a more local level would enable a multidisciplinary and multi-agency team, involving user representatives, to plan and evaluate service development creatively to meet actual health need. She further explained that she saw the nurse's role in the PCG/PCT as ensuring the PCG's/PCT's strategic plan and the health authority's HImP came from this 'grass roots' knowledge. This would enable the clinical team to be involved in both strategic and operational commissioning decisions and they would therefore have the opportunity to address health inequalities locally.

The skills nurses need

The previous analysis proposes a number of challenges which nurses must face if they are to actively contribute at both a strategic and operational level to the commissioning work of PCGs/PCTs. Box 3.3 illustrates the skills nurses involved in commissioning will need.

Addressing these challenges will be no mean feat, but with the introduction of PCGs/PCTs, nurses have been given the opportunity to fulfil their strategic contribution to health and articulate the expertise they bring to strategic decision making.

Box 3.3:   The skills nurses in commissioning will need

- a much broader political awareness, with the ability to translate the impact of public policy to nursing at the point of care delivery
- strategic skills, using the knowledge they have of the care of individuals within a population-focused commissioning framework
- language skills, to enable the integration of clinical knowledge with the public health corporate agenda
- the ability to manage the tension between professional and commissioning priorities, in order to be seen as able strategists who are primarily concerned with health gain for populations

Nurses have two particular strengths they bring to the commissioning process. The first is their relationship with the people they work with in the community, the networks they have across disciplines and organisational boundaries, and the knowledge they hold of the actual health and healthcare needs of the individuals they work with. The second is their potential ability to translate the knowledge they hold on the needs of individuals to the needs of populations within a local health strategy.

Whilst the first strength is self-evident, the second is underdeveloped. Nurses in PCGs/PCTs will require investment in acquiring strategic skills so that they can work between the clinical and the corporate, or put another way, the operational grass roots and the strategic if real change in the community's health is to happen. Of particular importance is the different approach which now needs to be taken to developing strategy. This 'grass roots' approach to strategy development should drive commissioning arrangements in the future and it is here where the strategic contribution of nurses can be made explicit.

It is important to clarify again that the strategic contribution nurses make to the commissioning process is broad, moving far beyond specialist concerns. Commissioning nurses operating strategically do not represent the specific interests of the nursing profession or a specialist group therein. They focus primarily on the health of the population and are able to translate the impact of decisions made for the population to the care of individuals. In reverse, nurses are also able to translate the impact of decisions made for individuals so that they make a difference for populations.

As one commissioning nurse explained to me, nurses empathise with individuals. They understand whether decisions made for the collective are meaningful to individuals. So nurses as strategists use both their operational and strategic knowledge to ensure that the decisions made by the PCG/PCT board make a positive difference to the life of people locally. Nurses contributing to commissioning decisions therefore focus their attention on collective health need and ground this in the experiences they have had caring for individual patients and the knowledge drawn from their clinical networks.

Research conducted with nurses working in commissioning has identified how nurses can use their clinical expertise to acquire new skills needed to operate effectively in a commissioning organisation. The example in Box 3.4 illustrates how this could be possible.

This example clearly illustrates how strategies and plans could be developed from the 'grass roots'. It is more complex than a top-down approach, for it involves engaging with the users of the service, and bringing about service changes for specific populations based on the needs they identify.

The skills nurses will need if they are to operate effectively in commissioning organisations include being:

- **a strategic thinker** who uses their 'grass roots expertise' in strategy development
- **a political operator**: a networker and an 'intelligence gatherer' who understands interpersonal politics and is able to translate public policy initiatives into nursing practice at the point of delivery, as well as influence public policy with the values held within nursing

Box 3.4:   Acquiring new skills

The nurse had recently moved to a health authority from a clinical role and was involved in a project developing services for childhood asthma. To develop her strategic skills she used her operational clinical knowledge to consider the care required by an individual child with asthma going into hospital through their A&E department. In so doing she designed and planned services according to her operational understanding of the healthcare needs of individual patients.

She used her clinical operational knowledge in a different way. She now considers the health needs of populations as defined by service users and in so doing views the service much more broadly than before. To keep her up to date with the views of users she has set up a user group of parents and children with asthma. The group has also informed her that they want direct access to the children's ward from their GP and not to have to go to A&E. They also want to know which GPs in their area have specialist knowledge of childhood asthma and they would like access to asthma specialist nurses.

- **a practice developer**: skilled at achieving clinical change
- **an organisational developer**: skilled at achieving organisational change
- **a manager of self**: confident, mature, reflexive, articulate, and able to deal with complexity and ambiguity.

The importance of commissioning healthcare services in the *New NHS* cannot be underestimated and has a number of implications for nurses. This chapter has outlined the major problems facing nurses as the new commissioning agenda takes hold. Nurses are being challenged to lift their sights from the operational delivery of care, where they are most comfortable, and to use their clinical knowledge within commissioning roles. By so doing, nurses will be contributing to a much broader strategic public health agenda. This shift to nurse strategist, however, will not prove easy.

It has been argued that the current policy climate provides new and exciting opportunities for nurses to develop their strategic understanding. Nurses on a PCG board or in the executive committee of a PCT can be involved in the production of a commissioning framework. The production of the HImP enables 'grass roots' health concerns to be integrated with political health priorities. Strategic leadership within nursing will, however, be essential if the interpretation between public policy and clinical practice is to be successful.[12]

It is clear that nurses are well placed to operate as 'grass roots' health strategists if they manage the challenges outlined within this chapter and acquire the necessary leadership skills. This means, however, a significant investment in leadership development so that a skilled cadre of nurse strategists are in a position to use their clinical knowledge to operate between policy and practice and contribute effectively to the nation's health.

References

1 Department of Health (1997) *The New NHS: modern, dependable.* The Stationery Office, London.
2 Department of Health (1997) *Designed to Care, Renewing the NHS in Scotland.* The Scottish Office, Edinburgh.
3 Department of Health (1998) *NHS Wales, Putting Patients First.* The Welsh Office, Cardiff.
4 Department of Health (1998) *Fit for the Future: a consultation document on the Government's proposals for the future of health and personal social services in Northern Ireland.* DHSS, Belfast.
5 Antrobus S and Brown S (1997) The impact of commissioning upon nursing practice: a proactive approach to influencing health policy. *Journal of Advanced Nursing.* 25(2): 309–15.
6 Light D (1998) *Effective Commissioning: beyond the NHS White Papers.* Office of Health Economics, London.
7 Royal College of Nursing (1996) *A Nurse on Board.* RCN, London.

8 Goodwin S (1992) Nurses and purchasing. *Senior Nurse*. **12**(6): 7–11.

9 Department of Health & Social Services (1983) *NHS Management Inquiry Report*. DA(83)(38) (The Griffiths Report). HMSO, London.

10 Huntington J (1993) Nursing a buyer's instinct. *Health Service Journal*. **28 October**: 19.

11 Strong P and Robinson J (1988) *New Model Management, Griffiths and the NHS*. NHS Policy Studies 3. Nursing Policy Studies Centre, University of Warwick.

12 Antrobus S and Kitson A (1999) Nurse leaders influencing and shaping health policy and nursing practice. *Journal of Advanced Nursing*. **March**.

Further reading

Antrobus S (1998) Board and lodgings. *Nursing Times*. **94**(50): 23–5.

4 PCGs: new roles for nurses

Sandra Rote

There seems little doubt that nurses are as competent to commission healthcare as any other professional group. On a smaller scale, nurses commission healthcare each time they plan the care of a patient, family or community. Given all the publicity and attention afforded to the nurse's role on a PCG board, it is interesting to ask 'why should nurses be involved in commissioning?'. Presumably, nurses only need to be involved if they can make a difference to healthcare, if their perspective can add to commissioning. This means nurses will have to be prepared to have a voice, to be independent and to say things which may conflict with other people's views. There is no valid reason for nurses being on PCG boards if they just want to maintain the *status quo*. As Sue Antrobus has argued in the previous chapter, nurses need to be contributing to commissioning decisions because their values and experience will ensure the decisions they make reflect local need and the services developed are needed within the community.

How can nurses use the structure of PCGs to influence the commissioning and provision of health services? Nurses can contribute to debates within the PCG about health needs assessment, evidence, effectiveness, health inequalities and multi-agency working.

The policy context

The health service reforms of the 1990s were hailed as a radical rethink of healthcare. The creation of the internal market was intended to overcome the financial problems inherent in the NHS by focusing on efficiency and effectiveness. It was thought market forces would reduce costs and improve services.[1] Most of those involved found it created competition and hostility between NHS trusts, health authorities and individual GP practices. Critics argued it created a two-tier system of healthcare and perpetuated inequalities in health.[2] The lessons learned from the experience of fundholding, locality commissioning and total purchasing were that GPs were able to commission services that were more sensitive to local needs than those commissioned by the health authority.[3] Providers were forced to change and improve services in order to ensure GPs continued to purchase them.

The White Paper, *The New NHS: modern, dependable*,[4] dissolved the internal market and replaced the GP fundholding scheme with PCGs. PCGs are based on configurations of GP practices which make up 'natural' communities. Each PCG has a board comprising GPs (four to seven), two community nurses, a social services representative, a lay member, a health authority non-executive and a chief executive. The PCG operates as a subcommittee of the health authority and is accountable to the health authority for its actions. As stated earlier, the services commissioned by the PCG have to take into account local need, existing services, available resources and national priorities. PCGs can progress to become PCTs, freestanding bodies responsible for commissioning hospital, community and primary care, and ultimately providing these services as well.

One of the fundamental differences with this new framework is the recognition that agencies outside of the NHS have an equal role to play in improving the health of the local population. NHS organisations are 'to work in partnership' with other organisations, such as local government and voluntary organisations. Each health authority is required to work with local NHS and non-NHS services to develop a HImP. This is a local plan of action to improve health and reduce inequalities in health.

Nurses in PCGs

The development of PCGs has given nurses the opportunity at long last to contribute to the commissioning and development of healthcare services. Over the last decade there have been very few nurses at an executive level who have been able to influence the commissioning of healthcare services,[2] and these are nurses who have been removed from clinical work – often for a long time. Most PCG board nurses, however, still have active caseloads and therefore are able to retain their clinical skills and knowledge, and use these to inform the commissioning process. Local knowledge of the area, the people and the environment will also ensure nurses on the board are well placed to articulate the needs of local people. Nurses will have different backgrounds and diverse knowledge bases, which will bring different values and perspectives from those held by other board members.

Although there has been much attention in the nursing media about the role played by board-level nurses, it is important to remember that all nurses have a role to play in the decisions made by the board. Nurses with specialist skills and knowledge will need to be co-opted on to the board and working groups to increase the breadth of knowledge available to the board and to spread the workload. It is vital that all nurses recognise their responsibility to support nurse board members and ensure that they are kept up to date about local events and service changes affecting people's health.

Nurses need to become more politically aware and use the influence they have carefully. Whilst their conduct and attitude during board meetings is important and skills such as assertiveness and negotiation are paramount, what happens outside the board meetings is of equal importance. The opportunity for influencing members of the board and working groups outside the main meeting should not be underestimated. Nurses may well find they can achieve more outside the meeting than they can during it.

Good communication skills will be vital to ensure nurses make the most of these opportunities. Nurses should develop a wide network of contacts to ensure they are up to date with current changes and developments and can share examples of good practice. It is well noted that nurses are able to use a wide variety of language styles, and this will be a particularly helpful skill at meetings.[5] Nurses are able to talk to members of the public in a way that can be understood, gaining an insight into the needs of the community.[6] This information will need to be presented to the PCG in a language they will understand. If nurse members are successful in doing this they will also be able to engage with the public and ensure the voice of service users are heard by the PCG board.

Nurses on PCG boards have a difficult role to perform. In their capacity as the nursing representative, they have to avoid focusing on one specific group of nurses, such as practice nursing. Their role is to articulate the views, experience, knowledge and values held within nursing. At the same time, the PCG board nurse needs to ensure she does not speak only when the board are discussing nursing issues. Nurses have a view about many issues affecting health, which come from their experience of working within the community. These views need to be clearly articulated, so the nurse is seen not as a 'nursing view' but as a 'health view'.

There is potential for a conflict of interest for nurses on the board. In one capacity they are employed either by a trust or

GP, but they also have a responsibility to take a corporate view when dealing with issues affecting the PCG. This means having to consider issues from the point of view of the PCG despite having an opposing personal view. This could become apparent when deciding which local NHS trust to buy services from or when making decisions about the distribution of services and staff in a practice where the GP is the nurse's employer. It is easy to see how a nurse could be put under pressure to take a particular view from her employers or colleagues. Nurses will need support from mentors to give them objective advice so that they service the interests of the PCG as a whole.

Organisational development

One of the challenges facing PCGs has been to develop (and nurture) a new organisation within a very short period of time. PCGs have needed to acquire the skills and organisational capacity to take on complex operational procedures such as needs assessment, commissioning services and clinical governance. Whilst for any new organisation this would be difficult, for PCGs the task is even more onerous. Other organisations are able to develop slowly and grow as the need and capacity arises, responding to external change and demand, and the change is incremental.

The timescale attached to the development of PCGs has meant that there has been very little time for the new organisation to evolve. Whilst some GPs have gained considerable management skills through GP fundholding and total purchasing, the majority have little experience in this area. In a short space of time GPs have had to develop organisational skills such as chairing board meetings and project management systems to lead the PCG. Whilst the chief executives may have many of these skills and can support the chair, it will be important for the chair to be seen by general practice locally to be influencing the management structure within the PCG.

Most PCG board members will have a mechanistic view of organisations, as this is how most NHS trusts, health authorities and local authorities operate. This view of organisations is apparent in the way people are managed, through hierarchical structures, rules, policies and procedures, which view individuals as part of the machine completing a process.[7] Nurses in particular have entrenched their practice in procedures, processes and rituals, for example consider the way the nursing process has been developed and applied. It could be argued that the volumes of manuals and guidelines are necessary to protect patients and promote individual patient care, but I would argue that these are not designed to benefit individuals, but to meet the organisational needs for risk management and outcomes. This mechanistic view can stifle practitioners, and thus prevent some individuals from being innovative. Such an approach also does not allow nurses to meet individual patient or local community needs.

During the first year when PCGs were being established and formal systems were not in place, life within a PCG felt chaotic, but at the same time practitioners were presented with new possibilities for changing services, structures and procedures. With the removal of traditional controls there is an opportunity to create an 'organic' organisation. Such an organisation evolves around the people in it, creating and adapting to the change, and eventually order will emerge naturally. Life is attracted to order and this can be achieved without having it imposed but by allowing flexibility and removing traditional boundaries. Order will come from finding out what works, the purpose of the organisation and its identity.

If this is allowed to happen, the resulting organisation will have the potential to develop the staff within it and be creative about the services and healthcare it provides. The organisation will also be able to value individual contributions, guide and support staff.

The key to creating order within an organic structure is ensuring everyone has access to information. Nurses will be vital for ensuring information is accessible to all, public and staff. However, for those used to working within a mechanistic organisation, the lack of control and chaos may feel frightening. For those who can seize the opportunity and adapt, the potential is there to be part of an open organisation which is proactive, responsive, cares for its staff and community, and is looking towards the future rather than the past.

PCGs commissioning healthcare services

The commissioning cycle is the process through which the board will have to go to achieve a rational basis for the commissioning decisions they make. The PCG will be expected to make strategic decisions about services for the whole population rather than on an individual basis. This process will replace the role previously undertaken by health authorities. The HImP is integral to this process and forms the basis for commissioning decisions. The framework, as set out in the previous chapter, essentially consists of four stages. These are:

- needs assessment
- setting priorities and objectives
- service implementation
- evaluation and review of progress.

The specific contribution nurses can make in each of the four stages is examined below.

Needs assessment

Before services can be commissioned, information needs to be gathered about the local community. This means collecting data and statistics for the whole population, not just from individual practices. Such data can be gathered in conjunction with the public health department related to age and sex of the population, mortality, morbidity incidence and prevalence of disease. Useful information can also be gained from a variety of other sources, such as hospital inpatient statistics and cancer registers. The distribution of diseases can highlight particular areas of need or disadvantage.[8]

In the past, there has been little integration between public health and primary care; primary care has focused on the individual whilst public health has focused on the population. More recently, closer links between public health and primary care have been promoted through an array of government policies such as HAZs. This more community-oriented approach can also be seen in the development of local HImPs. Input from PCGs in their first year has been limited; once they do become more involved and the process adopts a more community-oriented approach, community nurses will be able to play an important role in their development. Already, we have seen the appointment of a specialist health visitor to the post of HImP Co-ordinator (Devon and Plymouth Health Authority). A nurse's local knowledge will provide valuable insights into factors which affect the health of the population. This means not only considering health service provision but also local schooling, transport, shops, industry, housing and employment – all of which have a direct influence on people's health or how they perceive their health status.

Talking to local people can highlight health needs, such as fear of crime, lack of leisure facilities, inadequate transport, and inability to buy fresh fruit and vegetables. Whilst these factors may not be directly related to health service provision, they have an effect on people's health and their ability to lead a healthy lifestyle. For example, it is not helpful to encourage patients to eat wholemeal bread and skimmed milk if it is not available at local shops or is too expensive. In this situation, the nurse may decide the appropriate action to take to improve people's health is to work with the community and other agencies to lobby for better shops or a food co-op. Political action of this sort is not common within nursing. However, working with the community to improve conditions and services not only improves health but empowers the community to take action itself, which in turn raises the self-esteem and motivation of the community. This approach does not take power away from communities but increases their capacity to make changes for themselves.[9]

Health profiles maintained by community nurses will provide useful information on local services, gaps in current provision, specific health needs of small areas and factors affecting the local population.

Nurses are accustomed to working with a wealth of different agencies and involving self-help groups, whereas other members of the PCG board may not be used to this way of working and may find it threatening. It can be very challenging for a GP to acknowledge that other individuals and organisations should be involved in the commissioning of services. The medical model of health presented by the GP may be at odds with the view held by other members of the board. The challenge for board members is to educate one another about the different perspectives they hold on factors affecting health. Once a general understanding has been achieved about the contribution different agencies can make to health, then it will be possible to commission services that improve the health of the local population.

Nurses are now able to influence the commissioning agenda through the PCG. They can use the creation of these new organisations to shift the commissioning focus away from service delivery to client needs. Over the past ten years there has been a tendency within the NHS to continue to provide the same services because activity information has been collected which confirms the need for those services. PCGs need to focus on specific client groups (e.g. older people or children) rather than services. Using such an approach will allow new styles of services to be developed.

Setting priorities and objectives

Once information has been collected about the needs of the area and gaps in current provision have been identified, the PCG will need to decide which are the most important. Inevitably, more needs will be identified than the PCG has resources to commit. The PCG will need to take into account the national planning and priorities guidance (which, in 1998, for the first time specified joint priorities between health and social services). Decisions about priorities will be made after considering all the interventions available and the effectiveness of those interventions. To ensure non-medical interventions are also considered, nurses need to gather information from the research literature as well as service users about the efficacy, efficiency and effectiveness of non-medical interventions. There is evidence for non-medical interventions, such as the promotion of breast-feeding and parenting support groups, that the rationale for some developments will need to come from the community. Nurses will also need to develop and use local networks to gather information about what is happening within the community.

Nurses should consider using scenarios or vignettes to describe the outcomes of an intervention to a group of service users. Such a technique can be very powerful. Whilst one would not dispute the value of carefully researched and collected data, the real-life description of an event seen by a nurse can be very persuasive when trying to explain why certain services or ways of working are needed. Using this approach, nurses can explain the values fundamental to nursing and how they apply to practice. This approach is essentially client-focused rather than service-driven; however, the client could be a whole community.

Implementation

With GP fundholding, each practice had to negotiate and set contracts and service level agreements with each of their providers. GPs who chose not to hold a budget relied on the local health authority to undertake the process. The result was an enormous increase in paperwork and bureaucracy. To reduce the volume of bureaucracy the Labour government introduced Service and Financial Frameworks (SaFFs). The PCG now states the level and standards of the services they wish to commission, and the requirements of all PCGs are then combined by the health authority or a lead PCG into one block contract, which is then given to the provider units.

Within the SaFF there is the opportunity to develop services and change the way they are delivered, in conjunction with hospital and community trusts, to ensure the services are relevant to the community being served. For example, it may be important for a community to develop a community-based stroke rehabilitation service; this will only be achieved if PCG members work with the local acute and community trusts, social services and consumer organisations such as The Stroke Association. Again, nurses in the community are well placed to make contact with people from these different organisations to access information and feed this into debates to ensure that a new style of service is implemented. Engaging others also ensures that the implementation process is more successful.

By considering the needs of the whole population instead of individual people or practices, the needs of small, marginalised groups can be identified and met. Very often the needs of disadvantaged groups are not met, because their most urgent health needs are not medical or disease-focused. A change of emphasis towards a social or environmental model of health and the engagement of a wider number of organisations will facilitate the setting up of systems for tackling the wider influences on health. Lance Gardener (Chapter 5) and Jeni Bremner (Chapter 6) explore these issues further.

Reviewing progress

Evaluation of the services being commissioned provides the opportunity to reflect and consider how it could be done better. Standards and the quality of a service can be monitored and benchmarked against other services in other areas. Using waiting-list times as a marker of quality can result in some patients not going on a waiting list immediately or prioritising minor surgical procedures. Indicators such as wound healing time, lack of pressure sores or being able to talk to someone about their health would be more appropriate indicators of good care. Nurses have access to such information as well as other aspects of a service that patients value. This information needs to be fed into performance monitoring systems and used to inform subsequent commissioning cycles. Again, using such information will mean that nurses are influencing the health and healthcare agenda.

To the future and PCTs

It is a concern that at PCT level, the responsibility and strategic view required will result in nurses with clinical skills no longer being involved at board level. PCTs will need nurses with considerable management experience and time commitment to meet the organisation needs, and this is unlikely to be compatible with nurses who still have active caseloads. It will therefore be important for PCTs to ensure that there are adequate communication channels set up to allow nurses caring for patients to continue to contribute to the commissioning agenda.

PCTs will also provide new opportunities for nurses. For example, they will enable more joint working through the pooling of budgets and the deconstruction of organisational (and professional) barriers between trust-employed nurses and practice-employed nurses. This will facilitate the development of new services and more 'joined up' care for patients.

Conclusion

To ensure nursing is shaping the way policy is developing and evolving in a PCG (and PCT), as opposed to operationalising existing policy, nurses must become more vocal and be prepared to stand up for their beliefs and principles. This may be a daunting prospect; at times it will mean being the only voice against the common view of peers and contemporaries. Such a shift has to happen if nurses are to develop policies which reflect nursing's values of empowering, enabling, reflection and inclusivity. This means seeking to influence the way services are commissioned so they reflect these values, and gaining additional resources for public services seeking to achieve this.

Nurses will also have to challenge existing services and structures within nursing to ensure that they also reflect the values of nurses and nursing. This can be done at two levels, locally and nationally. Nurses must also be prepared to share and disseminate good innovative practice so that it can become part of the body of nursing knowledge. In this way, nursing theory and practice will develop and inform both the formulation and implementation of policy.

References

1   Levitt R, Wall A and Appleby J (1995) *The Reorganised Health Service*. Chapman & Hall, London.
2   Ham C and Shapiro J (1995) The future of fundholding. *British Medical Journal*. **310**: 1150–1.
3   Willis J (1992) Who needs fundholding? *Health Service Journal*. 30 **April**.
4   Department of Health (1997) *The New NHS: modern, dependable*. The Stationery Office, London.
5   King's Fund (1992) *The Professional Nursing Contribution to Purchasing*. NHSME Nursing Directorate, London.
6   Goodwin S (1995) Commissioning for health. *Health Visitor*. **68**: 16–18.
7   Morgan G (1998) *Images of Organization*. Sage Publications, Sacramento, CA.
8   Connelly J and Worth C (1997) *Making Sense of Public Health Medicine*. Radcliffe Medical Press, Oxford.
9   Freeman R, Gillam S, Shearin C *et al.* (1997) *Community Development and Involvement in Primary Care*. King's Fund, London.

Further reading

Hooker JC (1996) Nursing in commissioning: are we helping to build a stronger team? *Journal of Nursing Management*. **4**: 123–5.
Taylor P, Peckham S and Turton P (1998) *A Public Health Model of Primary Care: from concept to reality*. Public Health Alliance, Birmingham.

5 A nurse-led PCAP: 'just a mini-doctor?'

Lance Gardner

The Primary Care Act Pilot sites were the result of a major rethink by the Conservative government on how primary care was to be organised and delivered in the future. In June 1996, the then Secretary of State for Health, Stephen Dorrell, undertook what became widely known as the 'listening exercise'.

In a period when primary care was facing increasing demands from patients and low morale among staff as well as recruitment problems, Mr Dorrell realised that something fairly radical needed to be done if primary care was going to lead the NHS into the next millennium. To this end, Stephen Dorrell and Gerald Malone, the Health Minister, embarked on 60 meetings around the country, mainly with GPs, but also with nurses and other healthcare professionals, to seek their views on the way forward. As a result, the ministers were overwhelmed by the sheer volume of material they gathered. What they received was a collection of reasons why primary care was in its present turmoil, what the main problems were and many suggestions on how to solve them.

Mr Dorrell, to his credit, realised that there was not going to be one overriding solution that would fix all the problems within primary care. He therefore used the White Paper *Choice and Opportunity*[1] as a vehicle to enable primary care to solve some of its own ills. To this end, he invited GPs, GP practices and other stakeholders to identify the problems they faced which inhibited the development of high-quality primary care, along with the proposed solutions to these problems. If the Secretary of State felt that these proposals would demonstrate new opportunities for primary care, he would grant them pilot status for three years while they undertook to work in an innovative way.

This White Paper also provided opportunities for the private sector to enter the field of primary care delivery. This enraged the medical professional bodies and they used their political lobbyists to try to block this aspect of the White Paper at its first reading in the House of Commons. In this action they were successful. But in so doing, they thwarted many of the potential opportunities for nurses or others to put forward alternatives to 'GP-led primary care'.

In an effort to provide nurses with an opportunity to show what they could do, individual ministers, particularly in the House of Lords, began lobbying on behalf of the nursing profession to allow nurses to utilise the new legislation. What is interesting to note is that when the professional bodies that represent nursing began to look at the proposals that were beginning to be put forward by nurses under *Choice and Opportunity*, the majority required no legislative change whatsoever. For example, there were a number of projects proposed where nurses would deliver care in a branch surgery to patients registered with GPs in a larger centre. What these schemes needed was a change in attitude, particularly within the medical profession. Some would argue that the White Paper *Choice and Opportunity* was a focus for challenging traditional attitudes, particularly around the roles of doctors and nurses.

The drafted legislative framework that was produced following the publication of two White Papers, *Choice and Opportunity* and *Delivering the Future*,[2] did improve and favour new roles for nurses. The main catalyst for this shift was Labour's landslide win in the 1997 general election. The new Secretary of State for Health, Frank Dobson, believed that nurses have a unique role in the delivery of primary care, and went out of his way to encourage nurses to grasp the opportunities before them. To an extent, nurses worked at the central policy-making process in this instance. Nurses enlisted the support and enthusiasm of politicians and influenced the formulation of the NHS (Primary Care) Act 1997.[3] The remaining sections of this chapter focus on the development and implementation of a nurse-led PCAP pilot in Salford.

Salford nurse-led PCAP

A vacant practice list became available as a result of the untimely death of a 52-year-old single-handed GP, who had practised in the city for 29 years. The vacancy was originally advertised as a normal GP vacancy, and three doctors applied to take over the patient list and the premises. But the health authority saw the NHS (Primary Care) Act as an opportunity to try something different rather than maintaining the usual *status quo*. They asked the Secretary of State for Health to decide whether a traditional single-handed medical practitioner should be installed in the vacancy or whether a nurse should be given the opportunity to develop a PCAP site. 'The rest', as they say, 'is history'.

The pilot is based in what was once a dental surgery, deep in the heart of inner-city Salford, and very close to the real 'Coronation Street'. It is the only public building south of the M602 motorway, and approximately 2500 families live in close proximity. The standard mortality ratio for all causes is 150, and 208 for lung neoplasms, and there is almost total reliance on welfare benefits throughout adulthood. The major employment in the area is crime, and the resulting black economy thrives.

The practice team was 'adopted' in its entirety from the deceased GP. The administrative staff and the practice nurse are now employed by the pilot project. The district nurses and health visitor are shared with another practice locally, and remain employees of the local NHS community trust. The project nurse believed it was not in the best interests of nursing for him to feel it necessary to employ any nurses directly. I also believed it would create unwelcome hierarchy. As a result of this, the practice nurse is now employed by the community trust like all the other nurses in the team. The lead nurse is self-employed, and classed as an independent contractor just like a GP. The composition of the project team is listed in Box 5.1.

One unusual aspect to the organisation of this project is that it has purchased a 'package of support' from the local community trust. This package includes:

- human resources
- clinical support – both medical and nursing
- care-taking
- estate management
- domestic services.

The reason this agreement was developed is because it covers areas of practice management that GPs are traditionally very poor at, whereas community trusts have great skills and expertise in such areas. This advice and support has proved very worthwhile and has relieved a lot of the organisational burden from the practice.

Box 5.1:   The project team

- The lead nurse   full time – 60 + hours per week
- Part-time GP   20 hours per week
- Practice nurse   20 hours per week
- Practice manager   30 hours per week
- Three receptionists   2.0 whole-time equivalents
- Two counsellors   3 hours per week
- Health visitor   shared with another practice
- District nurses   shared with another practice

The ethos of the project

The Salford proposal was developed from a hypothesis in which it is believed that the health needs of communities in inner cities and socially deprived areas are intrinsically shaped by the physical and economic environment in which they live. If this is true, then the traditional biomedical role of GPs may sometimes be ineffective, whilst nurses can use skills and expertise in holistic care, and normalisation, which may be better suited to meeting the needs of such communities. This is not to say that there are not times and situations in healthcare when the biomedical model is not the right one for that individual at that time. In *Notes on Nursing* by Florence Nightingale (1863)[4] there is a fine definition of total care:

'...a human being to be nursed, a situation to be dealt with, its recurrence to be forestalled and, if possible, prevented. A patient's powers to be conserved while he was ill, he himself to be restored to *complete* health afterwards – in the modern phrase, rehabilitated, similar situations to be prevented in the future.'

In the majority of media coverage of general practice produced in this country, the problem of 'minor illness' or 'inappropriate use of the service' by the public is highlighted. Yet whilst nappy rash may seem minor to the highly skilled GP, it can be seriously disturbing and frightening to a single mum with no extended family nearby and a very fractious baby to care for. It is understandable that a significant percentage of the cases seen daily by a GP may seem 'inappropriate' to his/her skills, but they do feel very appropriate to a nurse. Many studies have attempted to assess the appropriateness of the GP's workload, and in 1986, Dr Julian Tudor-Hart, in his book *A New Kind of Doctor*,[5] stated that he believes 'that GPs spend 90% of their time using

10% of their skills'. The Salford-led PCAP project proposes that the same could not be said of many nurses, particularly in primary care.

The professional bodies representing GPs regularly complain about the volume of paperwork they are now expected to do. But in recognising that such an increase has taken place, is the GP best placed to meet that need? A significant percentage of that paperwork has a fundamental relationship to the level of welfare benefits a family may receive, and consequently the quality of housing, clothing and nutrition they can thereby afford. In a nurse-led PCAP the GPs do not do any paperwork which isn't related to clinical care, and nurses do the administration which relates directly to the patients' complete welfare. On some days, these nurses can spend more time with patients helping them to complete medical forms or doing Benefits Agency Assessments than they do on clinical issues. Is this a good use of their skills? I think it is – if a nurse can assist a patient to achieve some peace of mind about the roof over their head, or to know where the next meal for the children is coming from, the patient is less likely to attend a care centre on clinical grounds with anxiety, depression or, as is seen all too frequently, despair.

Some of the other nurse-led PCAP projects (n = 8) strive to provide services to those people in our communities who are often denied access to traditional GP-led primary care services. These groups include travellers, the homeless, refugees and those whose challenging behaviour is used as a barrier against them. Although people from these groups often experience ill health, which can be very specific to their individual style of living, many of their problems do not fit nicely into the pigeon-holes of traditional medicine. Their 'illnesses' are intertwined with the very individualistic way in which they seek to meet their activities of daily living. It could be said that the objective of medicine is to cure, whilst the nurse's aim is to care. I believe, however, that all healthcare professionals need to 'care' in their own particular way, and that those who choose to 'care' for vulnerable groups in society do so with an understanding that a 'cure' may not be the most appropriate outcome for some individuals, but a sense of wellbeing in such an individual would be a major achievement.

It is interesting to see how the nurse-led PCAP nurses as a group share a very similar set of beliefs and values despite the dissimilarity of the projects. They do not aim to cure but instead to care. They endeavour to be non-judgemental, and any bias that does exist tends to be in favour of the patient.

So what is so different?

First, the name. The project was determined not to be called a 'health centre' or a 'surgery'. After much trial and error, and soul-searching, the term 'care centre' was arrived at, because wanting to 'care' in our individualistic ways was the one value common to all the disciplines working on the project. The word 'centre' was used because it soon became apparent that the project was likely to become a natural focus for the local community. There are no other public buildings apart from two schools. There are two corner shops, no chemists, no community centre, no housing office and no other healthcare provision.

The project is endeavouring to provide services which are accessible to the community as a whole and not just practice list-centred. Ideally, the project would like patients to be registered with the project as an organisation rather than registering with the GP, but currently that is not allowable legally. Members of the community who may be registered with GPs elsewhere are welcome to use the centre or its services, and any relevant information will be passed on to their GP if they wish it to be.

Once the centre opened it soon became apparent that the

project team would have more social and non-NHS links than health service links. Social services saw the centre as something different and began to ask us to take patients who were receiving inappropriate or no primary care from other GPs in the city. These patients had care packages developed, care was shared and there was regular communication and co-operation between all those involved.

The local Citizens' Advice Bureau (CAB) began to ask for help in their role as patient advocates, particularly in tribunals over welfare benefits claims. It seems that most GPs in the city will not complete CAB health questionnaires about their patients because there is no payment involved. For reasons outlined elsewhere, the project sees their role in the welfare benefits system as crucial to optimising the wellbeing of the patients, and are therefore very happy to help the CAB to support the patient in any way it can.

Formal links are also being established with the two local primary schools in an effort to normalise health issues, so that children see them as 'good' and part of being 'well' rather than always linked to illness and perceived negatively. To this end, the children do projects based on health and come to the centre for guided tours as part of their orientation to their local community. Project team members give talks to small groups linked to their roles, and support teachers in their preparations for lessons on health-related topics. It is intended that the project will also assist the schools in health-related policy development in such areas as sexual health, personal development, management of medicines in school and sun protection. There are also plans to enable the children to paint murals in the care centre which will depict the kind of community in which they want to live in the future, so that they have something visual to strive for.

The problems or the challenges

What this nurse-led PCAP and others have done is to operation-alise a piece of legislation which wasn't originally aimed at their profession, and which they were not generally involved in developing. This has necessitated nurses having to mould a legal framework created for another profession so that nurses can deliver care in their way. As a consequence problems have occurred.

When the bid to become a PCAP was being developed, no one imagined that it would be the straightforward day-to-day issues which would raise the most problems. The most serious issue is that nurses do not count as an attending physician before a patient's death. This means that even if nurses from the team have cared for someone for days or weeks just prior to the patient's death, they can only confirm death but cannot sign a death certificate. Therefore, unless the GP is sent in to 'look' at the patient in the 14 days prior to the death, a postmortem will be required. This is necessary even if the GP is unable to make any meaningful contribution to the care the patient is receiving. Therefore nurses have to plan for a patient dying, and send the GP round to look at him or her just in case. This is obscene. Both the local coroner and the project nurse have brought this matter to the attention of the Secretary of State for Health, but he is powerless to do anything about it because death certifica-tion comes under the jurisdiction of the Home Secretary and is nothing to do with health. This issue has already had some very distressing consequences for the relatives of some of our deceased patients.

Another problem encountered by the nurse-led project is the signing of sick notes. Under the 1983 Medical Act[6] only hospital nurses can sign a MED 3 medical certificate, community nurses cannot. Apparently, this is because if a person is a hospital inpatient, he or she is obviously unfit to work. But the

MED 3 form is only the beginning of an administrative jungle of paperwork relating to welfare benefits, and many GPs do not have the time or inclination to give these documents the consideration and effort they deserve. Again, the Secretary of State for Health was informed, but welfare benefits come under the Benefits Agency, not the Department of Health, and so he was unable to help.

Within the NHS (Primary Care) Act 1997,[3] provision was made to enable GPs to take up salaried options if they so wished. However, because the pilots are only guaranteed for three years initially, it was felt that there were too many risks for the GPs' future financial viability. Therefore, clauses were written into the Act to ensure that the GPs' current occupational and financial situation was protected in the event of the pilot being discontinued. Unfortunately, this safety net does not exist for the two nurses who took self-employment in an effort to achieve PCAP status. One particular concern was that they would not be allowed to continue to contribute to the NHS superannuation scheme, and therefore their pensions would suffer in the long term. When this was brought to the Secretary of State's attention, he had a Statutory Instrument drawn up which made an exception to the law in the case of these two particular nurses so that they could continue to be part of the superannuation scheme. At least the Secretary of State was seen to act when he was in a rightful position to do so.

But at this point it became apparent how little nurses in general understand about how policy and legislation is created. If the Secretary of State for Health can draw up a Statutory Instrument for nurses to pay superannuation, surely he could do the same to allow nurses in PCAP projects to be allowed to sign sick notes or to prescribe. The author went through a very steep learning curve over the legislative process. Ministers, civil servants and learned members of the nursing profession all contributed to my understanding of the difference between primary legislation, secondary legislation and the powers of

MPs, Lords and Cabinet members to enact changes in legislation.

There has been an awful lot to learn, but it was necessary to enable the nurses within the PCAPs to understand the legislative process so that we could utilise it to our own advantage. Rather than just moaning about all the things that were wrong or difficult to overcome, as a group, the nurses involved in PCAPs began to use the system for themselves. It was decided that the nurse-led PCAP projects all faced 'challenges' rather than problems. Once recognised, these 'challenges' were then presented to ministers via local MPs, civil servants and the professional bodies representing nursing. The strategy was not to just moan about a problem, but to identify the challenge and then put forward our own solutions which would be acceptable within the legislative framework. In this way, the PCAP nurses were able to engage in the political process themselves in order to mould the legislation so that it would be more supportive to the nurse-led PCAP projects. This strategy also found favour among politicians because the nurses were bringing along their own solutions that were within the legislative framework. This made the politicians' jobs easier.

An example of this process can be found within nurse prescribing. The nurses working in PCAP sites were informed by a junior civil servant that under the 1992 Prescription by Nurses Act,[7] all nurses who wish to prescribe from the nurse formulary must be district nurses or health visitors, and must be employed by an NHS community trust or a GP fundholding practice. There was no leeway for nurses working in PCAP projects to be allowed to prescribe. The PCAP nurses launched a co-ordinated campaign to inform the nursing media, government ministers and the professional bodies of the problem, and suggested that the forthcoming Crown review or an amendment to the proposed NHS Act could be used as a vehicle to legitimise nurse prescribing rights for these nurses.

This process took six months, but in February 1999 the PCAP

nurses were informed that they would be allowed to become nurse prescribers under a planned amendment to the proposed NHS Act after lobbying from civil servants and the professional bodies on their behalf. At a meeting of the PCAPs nurses recently, a civil servant said:

> 'Do you realise what you have done? Ten nurses have persuaded the Government to alter legislation. This tiny group has managed to change the law of the land.'

The major benefits

Before the Salford Care Centre opened, the team were already experiencing the opportunistic nature of local criminals. They were helping themselves to equipment in the premises and staff cars. This led to a sense of vulnerability and a need to negotiate 'rights of passage' with local gang leaders. To this end, the lead nurse spent hours on the streets talking to local youths about what the project was trying to achieve and covertly trying to identify the influential gang leaders. There then followed some rather frightening encounters with the lead nurse turning up on the doorsteps of known 'professional' criminals and seeking their support for the project, and particularly the staff and their cars. What may surprise many people is that criminals do care. They have families of their own and value the efforts made by some healthcare professionals to try and help them. It could also be said that having highlighted them as 'leaders', they realised they had some responsibility to maintain the safety of the project and the team members. And this they are doing.

It often seems that because doctors and nurses have spent the majority of their training in large hospitals, they continue to cocoon themselves away from the community around them even when they move into working in primary care. Many healthcare centres or practices seem to have become large-scale 'fortresses of health', often indifferent and ignorant to the socio-economic environment in which their patients exist. There is much talk of health needs assessment, but in reality much of this is still very disease-focused, and the patients are rarely asked what they see as the health priorities locally. Invariably, when they are asked, they usually centre on pollution, housing and personal safety issues, which have little bearing on the 'targets' of most practices.

One of the key advantages of the PCAPs is that they are free to renegotiate these targets and are therefore not driven by cash-incentivised tasks. The pilots negotiate their financial packages with their local health authority a year in advance, and can therefore take a more 'complete' approach which seeks to fulfil the necessary disease-based targets and can also help the local community to meet its needs. An example of this is when a group of youths approached the project and asked if there was anything the team could do to get them a football pitch. They said they had nothing to do, and if they could at least play football they wouldn't get so bored and would probably commit less crime. The local community development worker was approached and he informed the local councillors of the request. The council asked whether the youths were trustworthy or capable of organising themselves properly.

The lead nurse and the community development worker organised a meeting between the youths and the councillors and other residents. The youths conducted themselves with a maturity and rationality which shocked all present, and as a result the council gave them a piece of land and their full support. Now the youths have formed themselves into 'Weaste Youth Action Group' and hold their meetings in the care centre, with the project supporting them with secretarial services and a treasury role. As a result of this apparent success, the group identified that the small children on the estate were in danger because they were always playing on the road. They have now developed their ideas for the football pitch to incorporate a safe play area for the small children, 'protected' by the teenagers. There are now plans to build a gym which will also include facilities for post-coronary rehabilitation and exercise on prescription. From the project perspective, this initiative has taken a little time and money but has had a fundamental effect on the youths because they are beginning to realise they have the power and ability to change their environment for the better.

Conclusion

Working with the local community has made it possible to engender a sense of 'mutuality' between the project and the local community. It could be said that this community is fortunate to have our project based in its midst, and they should be eternally grateful. But as a nurse-led PCAP, the project must see itself as being very fortunate to have been accepted by this community. The trust the people have unconditionally given to a nurse to keep them healthy when others around them have a GP is truly humbling, and makes this nurse feel very proud to be accepted as one of them.

Note: Primary Care Act Pilots are also known as Personal Medical Services Pilots. First wave PMS pilots can now choose to continue for a further two years.

References

1   Department of Health (1996) Choice and Opportunity. DoH, London.
2   Department of Health (1996) Delivering the Future. DoH, London.
3   Department of Health (1997) NHS (Primary Care) Act. DoH, London.

4   Nightingale F (1820–1910) *Notes on Nursing: what it is and what it is not* (new edn 1952). Duckworth, London.

5   Tudor-Hart J (1986) *A New Kind of Doctor.* Merlin Press, London.

6   Department of Health and Social Security (1983) *The Medical Act.* DoH, London.

7   Department of Health (1992) *Prescription by Nurses Act.* HMSO, London.

6 Nursing and Health Action Zones

Jeni Bremner

To make the links between nursing and Health Action Zones (HAZs) explicit, it is necessary to explore three issues: the philosophy of HAZs; the drivers for rethinking healthcare provision around the world; and what opportunities HAZs offer nursing.

In June 1997, the then Secretary of State for Health, Frank Dobson, launched the Health Action Zone concept at the NHS Confederation conference. HAZs were expected to overcome the fragmentation of the NHS brought about by the introduction of the purchaser/provider split and GP fundholding. HAZs were to be places where:

> '... all those involved in delivering the NHS on the ground would be brought together to develop a health strategy in co-operation with community groups, the voluntary sector, and local businesses. We envisage the Health Action Zones demonstrating the dynamism which is released when people and organisations are given the responsibility of working together to achieve agreed targets.'

HAZs cover geographical areas with high levels of deprivation. They explore mechanisms for breaking through the organisational boundaries with the aim of tackling inequalities and delivering better services and better healthcare. It is envisaged that although the NHS has a major role, other areas of central and local government also have a role in tackling factors that contribute to ill health. HAZ areas have been given additional funding for initiatives such as Healthy Living Centres and local community initiatives. HAZs are to be test beds for finding new ways of approaching and tackling old problems. They are to be places from which a new model of public service could potentially emerge. The additional funding given to HAZs is to enable them to modernise services and to tackle inequalities.

Each HAZ has adopted a different approach to tackling health inequalities, for example:

● Lambeth, Southwark and Lewisham are focusing on underage pregnancy, providing an integrated approach to child health and introducing a range of schemes to support families, including programmes to improve parenting skills
● Manchester, Salford and Trafford are focusing on developing integrated mental health services. This includes programmes to provide employment and training opportunities alongside improving mental health services.

In both of these examples, as in other HAZs, the goals will only be achieved through action within the NHS and outside the NHS, most notably local government. To provide integrated child health services, for example primary care, community, paediatrics, acute paediatrics, social services, local education authorities and schools need to work together to plan and deliver care. This is a huge task and will, in many cases, require a shift in professional attitudes.

If nurses are to make the most of the new opportunities offered to them under this new policy initiative of HAZs, they will need to understand and accommodate the dynamic nature of HAZs. They will need to be flexible, so perhaps most importantly they will need to develop new relationships and networks – and be able to look at the 'bigger picture'.

Modernising healthcare

The drive to modernise healthcare and to find more effective ways of delivering both health and social care is rooted in some of the challenges that are facing healthcare systems across the world. The key challenges are set out below.

Demographic changes

In the UK, there are an increasing number and proportion of citizens over the age of 65. Within this group of older people, the number of people over the age of 85 is also increasing.

Alongside these demographic changes, the birth rate is declining and women are choosing to start their families later in life. The inevitable consequence of these shifts is that the total societal burden of care is increasing as the total number of available informal carers is declining.

Families are increasingly fragmented. In the UK, 20% of families are single-parent families, and 42% of all marriages end in divorce. These families are often socially and economically disadvantaged. Many of the HAZ bids report a higher-than-average number of single-parent families. Some also have high numbers of older people living in the area.

Changes in the patterns of disease

One of the consequences of an ageing population is a change in the patterns of disease. In particular, there is likely to be an increase in chronic non-communicable disease. The World Health Organization (WHO) European Health Futurists Group predicts an increase in mental ill health, partly as a result of the expected increase in male long-term unemployment. It is likely that the pattern of new and resurgent infectious diseases, such as acquired immune deficiency syndrome (AIDS), will also continue.

There is a strong association between chronic illness and poverty. HAZs have populations with higher-than-average rates of chronic illness and mental ill health.

Changes in consumer expectations

The notion of choice has become embedded in our culture and this has shifted into peoples' mindsets and expectations about healthcare. The wider availability of information through the Internet and other media has led to an increasingly well-informed public who wish to engage more in a debate about treatment options.

This trend is likely to continue and will result in a different relationship between doctors, nurses and patients. This is also likely to be an increasing focus on self-care and disease management. Many of the HAZs have a priority to involve communities and service users more in decisions about local services.

Changes in work patterns

Changes in healthcare work patterns are already occurring. The shortage of nurses has led to a task-based substitution of health-care assistants for nurses. At the same time the drive to reduce costs has led to the extension of nurses' technical role and an increasing substitution of nurses for doctors.

In some specialties where there is a strong philosophy of multidisciplinary working, the boundaries between professional roles are becoming blurred. There is a danger that as we move more towards ambulatory care, the delivery of care in the home will lead to professionals increasingly working in isolation. Nurses and other professionals will need to develop effective communication channels and professional support structures.

There is the potential for HAZs to explore new models of

service provision and consider new roles for all healthcare professionals.

Changes in healthcare

Internationally, healthcare is moving towards shorter lengths of stay in hospital. Advances in medical technology are allowing healthcare to be delivered in an ambulatory and home-care setting. In the USA, hospitals are being built with no inpatient beds. A range of step-down and hotel facilities is being developed. Hospital bed usage consumes more resources than virtually any other intervention. However, social and psychological factors as well as primary diagnosis influence inpatient admission. Some HAZs are exploring how to prevent avoidable admissions and how to shift the emphasis of treatment to other community-based settings.

Opportunities for nursing in HAZs

HAZs are areas in the UK where changes in the style and delivery of healthcare potentially could be very rapid. The key thing that HAZs offer nursing is new opportunities – opportunities to experiment, to find new ways of delivering care, to begin to redefine their roles, and to find effective ways to develop and shape health policy.

The primary goal of HAZs, as stated earlier, is to tackle inequalities in health. They offer the people and communities involved the opportunity to reshape and redirect healthcare. The opportunity is there to shift the focus away from the reactive treatment of ill health to a broad proactive public health prevention agenda.

Many of the people living in HAZs are economically deprived and have complex social and health needs. One consequence of the increasing specialisation in the NHS and the drive towards ambulatory care is a separation of care from treatment. This leads to healthcare success being judged on the treatment outcome, rather than on the impact of the treatment on a person's life.

The consequence of the separation of care from treatment for nurses is to push nurses towards increasing levels of technical skills. Kitson, in an article in the *BMJ* in 1994,[1] articulates the dangers for nursing in pursuing a scientific route to win recognition and respect. She suggests that at the heart of nursing is 'the giving out and giving away of one's knowledge, skills and energies'. She goes on to suggest that professional nurses should work as community leaders and educators, equipping ordinary people with basic care skills.

HAZs are an opportunity to challenge this separation. People with complex needs are not well served by a fragmented healthcare system that has responsibility only for the treatment of a presenting medical condition. The sole pursuit of technological and scientific goals fails to recognise the realities of the lives of some of the most disadvantaged users of healthcare.

HAZs offer an opportunity for nursing to experiment with new ways of reintegrating treatment and care. There is a danger that moves to bring care and treatment together will be seen as a retrograde step. However, the world of healthcare has changed fundamentally in the past 20 years. It will not be a retrograde move if it increases the responsibility and autonomy of nurses. There is a need for different kinds of nurses, those with high levels of technical skill, those who are skilled carers and those who are both.

The nursing response to the possibilities of HAZs needs to be on a number of different levels. Nurses need time to think of, and develop, new models of service, both across professions and possibly across organisations. Nurses need to evaluate their impact on the communities they serve.

Developing new roles

Within HAZs nurses are already developing new roles. In the Tyne and Wear HAZ, a district nurse is seconded to work full time with the local authority housing department. The community mental health nurses are working with both patients and their families to maintain and enhance good mental health.

School nurses are running open-access sessions focusing on sexual health. In other HAZ areas, school nurses have been offered specialist mental health training to enable them to undertake early intervention work with young people who show behaviour problems. Nurses are also becoming involved in community development work.

There are numerous examples of this kind of innovative work focused on enhancing individual wellbeing and working with communities across organisational boundaries to foster health. The models are not exclusive to HAZs, but HAZs are areas where the government is looking at innovative models of public service.

Many of these initiatives are small and community-based. Seen alone they offer interesting models that may be replicated, but seen together they may offer the possibility of a new vision of nursing.

Developing new models

HAZs afford an opportunity to make explicit what nurses are doing in these areas. They also offer the chance to experiment with new models of nursing and, more importantly, to advertise the new models and bring to the attention of a wider audience the new directions that nursing is taking.

HAZs also offer the opportunity for nurses to develop and pilot new career structures and to explore the constraints that are preventing nurses pushing forward the boundaries. What are the consequences for nurses who go and work in non-NHS organisations? How does nursing recognise and value the contributions that those nurses make? For example, does the current grading and career structure support or hinder nurses exploring new roles?

A HAZ could potentially request a legislative freedom that would enable the development of nursing. Can nurses offer a united view of what they would ask for? I suggest that the new models and the extension of the nursing role that is taking place in these communities are crucial to the development of nursing as a profession. They demonstrate nurses taking leadership and breaking new ground in their care for their communities.

Within HAZs, the public health role of the nurse can be explored further, but it must also be described. Nursing must not miss this opportunity to describe its emergence. Nursing must not be tempted only down the path of managed care and doctor–nurse substitution. That is a valid route for some nurses but not for nursing. We must seek to build evidence and demonstrate that the process of care and the experience of being cared for are the elements that can reshape and refocus our healthcare system.

As new models develop, nurses need to organise and plan strategically to take advantage of the possibilities that HAZs offer. If HAZs are where new models of public service are going to be shaped and developed, then nurses need to be actively involved, shaping the models, making sure that they are able to influence the opinion formers and the developing agenda. Nurses need to be able to influence and shape the new public service *Zeitgeist*. This will not only take place in HAZs, it will also take place at a national and a regional level. However, within HAZs there are freedoms and possibilities available to nurses now to allow them to shape the agenda.

This challenge is not easy. The voice of nursing has often struggled to be heard.

Influencing policy

Most healthcare, and indeed most public sector, workers spend most of their time examining:

- what they are doing
- what they could be doing
- what they should be doing.

Generally, most attention is given to what we (nurses) are doing rather than what we should be doing. There is rarely enough time to think creatively about what we could be doing. Nursing needs to express what it could do, and there is not one but many answers.

Nurse leaders therefore need to encourage and support nurses in exploring what they could be doing. Ideally, nurse leaders should come from many different areas within the profession and work at different levels in different areas. If we, as nurses, sat down and thought about the problems facing healthcare and the challenge of tackling health inequalities, what solutions would we come up with?

Nurses and nursing need to use the opportunity offered by HAZs. Nurses need to be able to use their knowledge and describe these new directions to nursing. We need to make sure that nurses working with HAZs are encouraged to think about what they *could* do. We need to make sure that they are engaging with, and beginning to influence, the way new models of public service develop.

New models of public service might not talk directly about nursing but they will be enriched by the contribution and thinking of nurses. Our training as nurses helps shape the way we think about the delivery of healthcare. We must not allow nursing to be sidelined in this debate.

In 1994, Kitson[1] was arguing that:

'Nursing needs to demonstrate its commitment through innovative schemes that bring together its essential ingredients – empowering, enabling and educating people to take control of their lives.'

HAZs offer nurses the opportunity to innovate, evaluate and advertise what nursing has to offer. This is an opportunity that nursing cannot afford to miss.

Reference

1   Kitson A (1996) Does nursing have a future? *BMJ*. **313**: 1647–51.

7 Public health policy: the European dimension

Susan Williams

'Europe' means different things to different people. This chapter focuses on the European Union (EU), a fairly narrowly defined 'Europe' of 15 member countries, which is, however, likely to expand almost twofold over the next decade. Compared with organisations such as the World Health Organization, the EU is a relative latecomer to developing an explicit public health policy. Partly for this reason, but also due to the EU's enormous impact on UK economic and social policies, developing a nursing perspective on EU policies within the public health sphere represents an important challenge.

This chapter will look at the way in which the European Community (EC), later becoming the EU, has influenced public health in the UK and how an explicit public health policy is only just beginning to emerge. I will then look at some of the challenges for developing a nursing perspective to this policy process.

The policy development process at EU level

To understand why public health policy has been slow to develop at European level and why this whole process may seem at first sight both impenetrable and irrelevant to nursing, it is important to look at the way the EU operates and the principles by which it was established and has developed. These form the backdrop to the EU's public health activities today and the opportunities for shaping them.

The EU's remit is very strictly defined and specified in the Treaties. It cannot act in areas where it has not been given a specific mandate to do so. Over time, its competencies have been broadened with moves towards greater European integration. But such moves have often highlighted the constant tension which exists between member states' views of what is their own business and which areas of policy development they will share with European institutions. As we will see in later discussions, this is one of the reasons for the late development of a public health policy at EU level.

European decision making is one stage removed from national implementation and even further from 'grass roots' implementation. The EU institutions are very aware that they are perceived as distant, irrelevant or interfering, and there has been a strong push over the past five years to bring Europe 'closer to its citizens'.

Formally, the decision-making system gives member state governments the final say in most decisions, but the European Commission (the nearest equivalent to the civil service) has the unique right to initiate policy and proposals. These are then scrutinised by advisory bodies and the European Parliament (the only directly elected EU body), which has played a much greater role over the years – using its democratic legitimacy to argue for more power.

There is no elected 'government' at EU level which can push through its own agenda for action. Decisions are generally reached by 'consensus' both in the European Parliament and in the Council of Ministers (made up of ministers from each member state government), rather than adopting the adversarial approach of the UK parliamentary system.

The European Commission is a key player in policy development because it is the main initiator of proposals and guides these proposals through the decision-making process. But it is very small and compartmentalised into separate Directorates General (DGs) with their own conflicting interests. It needs expertise from outside its administration to develop initiatives in the wide range of areas within its responsibility. It is therefore very open to interest groups, particularly if they are pan-European and can provide reliable information, research, networks and feedback from across member states at the level of policy implementation. This has led to the growth of a whole lobbying apparatus in Brussels around the Commission and the Parliament – sometimes known as the Eurosphere. In the early days lobbying came predominantly from industrial interests, particularly the agri-industry lobby, but also pharmaceuticals and the tobacco industry. Over the years, a strong environmental and consumer lobby has emerged and more recently a public health lobby.

All this shows that the policy development process is, as ever, a complex one, summed up succinctly as a 'vast, proliferating range of groups, conflicting national interests, a strongly sectorised but small bureaucracy, unpredictable agendas and changing decision rules'.[1]

Europe's impact on public health: the early days

The European Economic Community (EEC) was established in 1957, the UK joining much later, in 1973. The EEC was established essentially as a customs union in which there would be free movement of goods, services, capital and people.

Whilst some progress was made towards achieving this common market, many trade barriers remained and in 1986 the member countries agreed the Single European Act, designed to speed up the whole process with over 250 legislative measures which would herald the creation of the single market by the end of 1992. Governments saw the single market almost exclusively in terms of a free trade area and the then prime minister, Margaret Thatcher, signed up enthusiastically. Any social legislation, on the other hand, would hinder its development. But other governments argued that the 1992 project should not be limited to economic concerns. Free movement of workers required some guarantee of minimum standards in the workplace, and any remaining barriers to free movement of people and all that went with it should be removed. This included reciprocal arrangements for social security and emergency healthcare.

To this end, in 1989, all member governments, except the UK, signed the Social Charter,[2] which set out a range of basic employment rights. It was a solemn declaration without the binding force of law, but the signatories were morally and politically committed to upholding the social rights it contained. It included commitments to improving living and working conditions and health and safety in the workplace. But it did also go further in covering people who for one reason or another were not active in the labour market. Its principles envisaged, for example, that those unable to work should receive sufficient resources and social assistance. Nevertheless social policy remained predominantly labour market policy rather than social welfare policy for the EC's citizens.

From the action programme which followed on from the Social Charter came the first proposals for legislation for the protection of pregnant women, rights for part-time workers and the working time directive. The UK government saw such social legislation as undermining business and the free market and questioned whether some issues were really part of the EU's remit at all.

The Social Chapter,[3] which the UK also refused to sign, was born out of the Charter and was agreed in 1991. The Labour government, when it took office in May 1997, agreed that the UK would accede to the Social Chapter, making it an integral part of the EU's activities.

The second half of the 1990s saw a new mood in economic and social policies, with growing unemployment in Europe and fears about its competitiveness in an increasingly global market. European social policy has continued a firm commitment to social solidarity and preventing social exclusion but also expressed the need for adaptability and flexibility in the labour market, coupled with lifelong learning, to help Europe remain competitive with the rest of the world.

There is now a marked convergence between the aspirations of European social policy and the UK government's approach in its domestic employment agenda with a growing recognition of the need to promote 'employability', 'an inclusive society' and 'flexibility' to meet the challenges of the 21st century.[4]

So the EU has a long-standing interest in social policy in relation to employment and has had a major impact in the UK on working conditions, particularly equal opportunities for women and health and safety in the workplace, predominantly through legislation but also through funding for employment programmes as part of its regional policy. The EU has not ignored totally issues of poverty, inequalities, 'social exclusion' and disadvantage, but these are areas where member governments have been extremely sensitive about the prime role of national governments rather than the European institutions in tackling such problems.

Public health

From the very beginning the EC's remit included within its provisions the ability to restrict the import and export of goods to protect human health. These provisions were later strengthened with the Single European Act which stated that measures taken to create this single market should 'take a high level of health protection as a base ... in the field of health, safety, environmental protection and consumer protection'.[5]

The main emphasis was therefore on control and protection from environmental and workplace hazards as part of ensuring a 'level playing field' for business in the single market. Many other areas of health have been affected by the moves towards a single market. These include minimum standards in the training of doctors, nurses and other health professionals, or for regulating medicines, medical devices, dangerous substances, etc. So whilst for the first 35 years of its existence the EC had no remit for public health, it has nevertheless had a major impact, both positive and negative. Health concerns were dealt with within the context of fostering economic development, particularly in the poorer regions of the EU, supporting Europe's agricultural policy and creating the single market. These priorities obviously conflicted at times with the health needs of the European population.

Towards an EU public health policy? The Maastricht Treaty

The year 1991 was to herald a new era in EU public health activity. In one of their periodic reviews of the EU's treaties which clarify its remit, member state governments agreed at Maastricht that the EU should be given a specific competence in 'public health'.

The agreement came about for a number of reasons.[6] It was partly by stealth, in that the European Commission had already begun to run specific health promotion programmes through its Europe Against Cancer and Europe Against AIDS programmes. There had also been a move for some time towards preventive measures in other areas as well, such as protection of the consumer and the environment, both of which were strengthened in the Maastricht Treaty, along with health. Giving a focus to this activity and legitimising it – as well as limiting it to areas which were worth pursuing at European level – was the next logical step.

The Maastricht Treaty also came at a time of growing economic, monetary and political integration, when the EU's role was expanding in relation to member governments. This was coupled with a desire by the European institutions to show how Europe directly benefited its citizens (and voters!). The European Parliament was pressing for a greater say in decision making at EU level and therefore supported new remits where it would also have the power to make joint decisions with the Council of Ministers.

The wider European health lobby did not really develop effectively until after the Maastricht Treaty, although individual groups lobbied for inclusion of a public health article in the Treaty and for a role in the implementation of the new public health competence.[6,7]

So Article 129 of the Maastricht Treaty – the public health article – contained three key elements:[8]

- that the Community contributes to a high level of human health protection by encouraging co-operation between member states
- that its actions should concentrate on prevention of disease, particularly major health scourges, by promoting research into their causes and transmission and by promoting health information and education
- that health protection requirements should form a constituent part of the Community's other policies.

In doing all of these, Article 129 stresses that the European Commission must work with member countries in co-ordinating their policies and programmes and it specifically rules out any harmonisation of laws and regulations across member states. The emphasis is on prevention rather than treatment and care, and the Article *permits* rather than *enforces* and allows fairly wide scope for interpretation.

Public health is not defined and it would be fair to say that its meaning is understood differently in EU member countries. Particular countries' pet topics or concerns are also included rather than restricting the remit to an overall framework. So, for example, specific reference was made to drug abuse due to pressure from the Italian government. The reference to excluding harmonisation of legislation is believed to have been included to keep the UK on board, after they had argued that the structure and delivery of health services was a national and not a European issue.[6]

The Commission was left with a rather ill-defined role and set about issuing a consultation document – a Commission Communication – which represented the first tentative steps towards some kind of public health strategy.[9]

This 1993 Communication described the major health issues

in Europe and proposed criteria for determining what the EU's priorities should be, as well as suggesting a number of action programmes.

The criteria proposed focused on identifying diseases or conditions suitable for action at European level, such as:

- diseases which cause premature death or high death rates
- diseases which cause high morbidity or serious disability
- preventable diseases
- those diseases that have a detrimental effect on quality of life or on the economy or society (e.g. high absenteeism).

What emerged from this was a set of separate funding programmes to cover most of the main areas identified, which represented a predominantly disease-focused, medicalised approach to public health. Some of the programmes have still not been fully implemented today, which makes any review of their impact quite difficult. The programmes cover:

- cancer
- drug dependency
- health promotion, education and training
- AIDS and certain other communicable diseases
- health data and indicators
- monitoring and surveillance of communicable diseases
- intentional and unintentional accidents and injuries
- pollution-related diseases
- rare diseases.

In practice, this has meant that implementation of the 'public health policy' focuses around a series of programmes which fund individual projects from organisations/networks who decide to apply. Whilst each programme has a set of funding criteria, there are no overall strategic objectives. Nursing groups have received funding from a number of these programmes for their activities, such as the cancer programme and the AIDS and health promotion programmes. But this is a very fragmented form of policy implementation and there is no evidence that feedback is sought and channelled to influence future policy.

According to a recent report commissioned by the European Parliament, there are some larger-scale projects which deal with issues that can be done better at a European/international level, including the communicable disease surveillance networks, a European investigation into cancer and nutrition, and work on the epidemiology of substance abuse. Apart from well-designed projects which were clear about their strategic goals, the other reasons for their effectiveness and added value were their good sample size, standardised data and ability to test hypotheses relating to the geographical diversity of the EU.[10]

The public health programmes are administered from the Public Health Unit, a part of the Directorate General for Employment, Industrial Relations and Social Affairs (DGV) of the European Commission, which is one of more than 20 DGs of the European Commission.

Whilst the approach has been criticised as unimaginative and not fully exploiting all the opportunities provided by the new public health article, the Commission has also been aware that health issues are very sensitive ones. Policies in this field risk being caught in the interplay between health systems and values based on very different national traditions and the legitimate role of the EU in areas where it can 'add value' to national activity.

To integrate health protection requirements better into other European policies, the Commission created an inter-service group with representatives from all the DGs with a health interest, and began producing an annual report on work undertaken in other policy fields. But the Public Health Unit remains small, with little power of influence, and at a distance – in Luxembourg – from the rest of the European Commission, and has its own DG for social affairs in Brussels. Public health activity has generally had a low profile both within the European institutions and amongst health professionals in member state countries.

If this has changed at all over the past couple of years, it has been above all because of a major European public health scare – bovine spongiform encephalopathy (BSE).

Strengthening the public health remit:

Amsterdam and beyond

The first openings for public health action defined in the Maastricht Treaty were seen by many as just a first stage and they looked forward to further development at the next Intergovernmental Conference in 1996 to review European integration and draft the Amsterdam Treaty.

The Amsterdam Summit of Heads of Government was held after a period of great scepticism about what Europe really did for its people. There was a feeling that Brussels was interfering in everything but without any positive gains. There were concerns over Economic and Monetary Union (EMU) convergence criteria, cuts in public spending and jobs, as well as wider international issues such as the EU's ineffectiveness in a war on its doorstep in Bosnia. For this reason the Amsterdam Treaty was packaged so that it was seen to be addressing people's major concerns: unemployment, individual rights, security and protection from crime. This meant that any great expansion of the EU's powers was ruled out and there was even talk of 'repatriation' of certain policy areas.[11]

Then came the BSE crisis. This set the scene for a serious reappraisal of the way in which the European Commission and member states, particularly the UK, protected human health.

More than anything, it created a growing awareness of the needs and problems of public health in Europe and demonstrated the conflict between public health and commercial interests. It highlighted the fact that a 'high level of human health protection' had not been applied to decisions made in relation to agricultural policy.

As a result, certain scientific committees dealing with animal and plant health which were situated in the DG for Agriculture within the European Commission were moved to a new, expanded DG for Consumer Protection. The European Parliament was given a greater say in issues relating to veterinary and plant health measures, and health ministers rather than agriculture ministers were given the lead on such matters. The EU also committed itself to taking consumer protection requirements into account in drawing up and implementing its other policies.

In addition, the commitment to ensuring that health protection is taken into account in other Community policies has been strengthened in the Amsterdam Treaty. This paves the way for a more strategic multisectoral approach to addressing public health issues and shifts the emphasis away from a medical model as it also requires a multidisciplinary approach in transport, environment, economic regeneration and agricultural policy. The Treaty shifts the wording to emphasise its aim is to *improve* health rather than *prevent* disease.

The Treaty update did not escape influence from specific member states' key concerns. Minimum requirements have been added in respect of the quality and safety of transplant organs and substances of human origin, blood and blood derivatives across Europe. This was an issue of particular concern to the Dutch, who hosted the summit and held the presidency of the EU at the time the Amsterdam Treaty was being negotiated.

The health lobby was disappointed about the final outcome, which it felt did not improve the public health article significantly and concentrated predominantly on the issues raised in the BSE crisis. An opportunity was lost for a radical overhaul to improve EU contribution to public health in Europe.[12] But there was little desire for radical change by governments and, perhaps on the positive side, it helped to clarify what member governments did and did not want.[11]

The present public health programmes will come to an end soon. The Treaties have been revised to extend slightly the EU's remit, and the EU must also begin to prepare for its expansion to the East. For these reasons, and in recognition of the changing health challenges European countries face, the European Commission issued a new proposed framework for Community public health policy in 1998 to look at 2000 and beyond.[13]

The Commission's proposed framework suggests that the EU concentrates on three core areas of activity in future:

- improving information for developing public health (trends in health status, health determinants, tracking health system developments)
- reacting rapidly to health threats (surveillance, early warning and rapid reaction systems, particularly for communicable diseases)
- tackling health determinants through health promotion and disease prevention (one action programme focusing on health determinants such as nutrition, etc.).

This means streamlining the present public health programmes. Most significantly it opens the way for a much broader approach to the determinants of health, including socioeconomic factors and the opportunity to do something more effective to integrate health protection into other EU policies.

Health organisations and the European Parliament have been lobbying for the European Commission's main priority to be the introduction of health impact assessment for use in all its proposed activities.[14] It has been estimated that at least 12 of the European Commission's DGs deal with health-related issues.[15] A particularly crass example of divergence in policies is the EU's anti-cancer work, its restriction of tobacco advertising and labelling, but its continuing support, through the Common Agricultural Policy, to tobacco growers in southern Europe.

So a definite shift is taking place towards a set of public health objectives which reflect more closely the way that nurses work in the public health arena. There is a shift away from disease-focused programmes, a recognition that a key focus should be on multidisciplinary work to promote health across a whole range of policies which are implemented by different agencies – government, local authorities, industry, farmers, communities, etc. However, the very nature of EU activity and the need for it to concentrate on areas where it can add value to local, regional and national activity, as well as the physical distance of its institutions from the level of practice, means it is often difficult to see the link between policy and implementation. Added to this, the continued weakness of EU structures to push public health higher up the agenda and the lack of public health expertise in the European Commission contribute to it remaining a marginalised area of influence.

A policy for nursing?

The overarching theme of this book is to look at the way in which policy development can be influenced by the way in which nurses alter policy by putting it into practice. Up to now this chapter has said very little about nursing, since, to be blunt, nursing does not feature strongly in EU public health policy.

Within the EU context, nursing has hardly begun to grasp the public health agenda and even recognise the impact that it has. This may be because this impact is filtered through national processes – for implementing EU legislation on the environment, on working conditions or on food safety, for example. Or it may be because EU public health policy implementation is piecemeal and does not represent a policy at all but exchange of ideas and experience, for example activities funded by the public health programmes. Or the impact may arise from policy not associated with health and therefore not perceived as part of nursing policy, for example EU employment and regional development policies.

There is also much for the policy makers at EU level to grasp in relation to nursing. Since the European institutions work within the context of 15 different member countries, the view of nursing within the Commission, Parliament and Council of Ministers will be influenced by the status of nursing in different member countries and the ability of nursing's representative bodies to influence national policies in their own countries. It is possible that with the entry of Finland and Sweden into the EU in 1995, both the vision of public health and the key role of nursing may have been strengthened.

If this is the general picture today, it does not mean that there are not opportunities in the next few years for nursing to have a greater impact on the way the EU public health agenda operates.

Some thoughts and challenges for the future

Nursing groups have participated in some of the funding programmes, but there is a need to encourage a strategic link between the outcomes and future policy work. One project is underway at present, funded by the European Commission and co-ordinated by the Standing Committee of Nurses of the EU, to look at developing a programme of education for nurses in public health across the EU. Although only in its early stages, potentially this project offers the possibility of demonstrating the key nursing role in public health and the contribution it can make to further develop public health policy.

Integration of health protection requirements is not yet embedded in Commission work. The main focus of the EU remains economic (monetary union, employment, single market), and public health concerns are not always compatible with these overriding aims. The recent recognition of the need for practical tools to introduce health impact assessment offers an opportunity to develop methodologies which take a much wider approach to public health. Again the European Commission is dependent on external expertise to pursue this agenda. Nurses need to be showing and developing their skills to assist in this process.

Until recently there was no strong political figure at Commissioner level with sole responsibility for promoting the importance of health matters. This meant that nursing not only needed to understand better the work of the one small Public Health Unit and offer expertise, but also to make links and champion its role in public health with other parts of the European Commission and Parliament. This means developing links with officials and politicians who will not necessarily recognise the link between what they do and public health interests.

In 1999, the European Commission was significantly restructured. David Byrne was appointed as Commissioner for Health and Consumer Protection and this may well result in a more co-ordinated approach to health matters in the EU.

The health lobby may have much to learn from developments in the environmental field. The EU has always had much greater powers in the field of environmental protection than have been granted it under the public health provisions. Environmental protection has now become one of the main objectives of Community policy with a view to promoting sustainable development. The Commission and the member states must prepare environmental impact assessment studies when they make proposals that are likely to have a significant effect on the environment, although some commentators are not convinced that integration of environmental objectives has really been achieved yet.[10]

Local government also has a long history of involvement and influence in Europe and has been a key player in the EU's regional policy and funding for many years. There is a suggestion by the European Parliament that a potential area of interest to future EU public health activities could be to look at the development of a regionally based health policy.[14] This provides further opportunities for collaboration with local government agencies and more direct involvement in implementation. With the advent of regional development agencies and regional assemblies in England and assemblies for Scotland, Wales and Northern Ireland, roles in relation to Europe also look set for a shake-up.

The European Commission is very open to suggestions/information from lobbying groups, but any proposals it submits have to reflect the diverse cultures of the member states and the relative importance (and interpretation) of public health. The north/south divide became very obvious in the debate on implementing the first set of public health programmes with southern countries seeking disease-specific programmes and the northern countries looking at more horizontal issues, such as data collection, monitoring and surveillance of communicable diseases, etc. There seems to be a greater acceptance for the next series of programmes that the EU should focus on health determinants and information gathering rather than diseases. This means that the type of funding available will be more open to the types of activities that nurses are involved in, providing that they are also able to link strategic and local activity.

So there are exciting times ahead, and with nurses often proving to be excellent networkers and alliance builders, there are many possibilities for them to co-operate with other agencies and begin to develop a stronger input to implementing policy more directly and to help in shaping it.

References

1   Mazey S and Richardson J (eds) (1993) *Lobbying in the European Community*. Oxford University Press, Oxford.
2   Community Charter of the Fundamental Social Rights of Workers (1989), Commission of the European Communities, Luxemburg.
3   Protocol on Social Policy. In Beaumont P and Moir G (1994) *The European Communities (Amendment) Act 1993: text and commentary*. Sweet and Maxwell, London.
4   Labour Party (1998) *Europe: policy paper*. Labour Party, London.
5   Single European Act. In Beaumont P and Moir G (1994) *The European Communities (Amendment) Act 1993: text and commentary*. Sweet and Maxwell, London.
6   Toward S (1995) *The Impact of European Integration on the National Health Service and on Health Policy*. Occasional paper. University of Southampton.
7   Standing Committee of Nurses of the EC (1993) *The Nurse's Contribution to EC Public Health Policy*. Standing Committee of Nurses of the EC, Brussels.
8   Treaty on European Union. In Beaumont P and Moir G (1994) *The European Communities (Amendment) Act 1993: text and commentary*. Sweet and Maxwell, London.
9   Commission of the European Communities (1993) *Commission Communication on the framework for action in the field of public health*. Office for Official Publications of the European Communities, Luxemburg.
10 European Parliament Directorate General for Research (1998) *European Union Health Policy on the Eve of the Millennium*. European Parliament, Strasbourg.
11 Stein H (1997) *Eurohealth*. 3(2): 4–8.
12 Williams S (1995) *Eurohealth*. 1(3): 28–30.
13 Commission of the European Communities (1998) *Communication on the Development of Public Health Policy in the European Community*. Commission of the European Communities, Luxemburg.
14 Needle C (rapporteur) (1999) *Report on the Commission Communication on the Development of Public Health Policy in the European Community*. European Parliament, Strasbourg.
15 Chambers G (1996) *Eurohealth*. 2(3): 7–11.

8 Towards a policy for nursing

Nicola Walsh and Pippa Gough

This book began by suggesting that we should move beyond a policy analysis *of* nursing towards a policy *for* nursing. We argued that nurses' knowledge and experiences of patients and their needs could make an essential contribution to the development of policy. So, how can nurses become more involved in the policy-making process, in particular policies that improve the health of the population as well as the individual? What knowledge, skills and experience are needed so that nurses can articulate what they do on a day-to-day basis and feed this into the formulation of policy?

The specific focus of this book is on the development of public health within the current NHS reforms and the EU. Each of our contributors has set out ways in which nurses and nursing could (and are) shape(ing) the development of policy in this area. Some of the chapters, such as those written by Jane Naish, Sue Antrobus and Susan Williams, offer the reader a more theoretical viewpoint as to how it might be done, whilst those by Lance Gardener and Sandra Rote offer the reader a 'rich story' of experience. Themes that are common to all include: the marginalisation and visibility of nurses; the need to develop relationships and networks, and to think beyond one's current role; and the need for a solution-focused approach.

Marginalisation and visibility

This is a recurrent theme emerging from all of the six chapters. Taking a historical perspective, Jane Naish clearly illustrates how nurses and nursing have been marginalised from the public health structures within the NHS. This is not to dwell on the notion of 'nurses as victims', however, but rather to emphasise the possibilities for nurses to take their place and seize the new opportunities being presented to them through the emergence of new organisational forms such as PCGs/PCTs, HAZs and PCAPs.

With new posts and new roles, nurses can achieve a 'presence' at the policy high table. Nurses need to ensure that they contribute to discussions that fall beyond nursing-specific issues. The views of nurses should not be seen by others as just giving the *nursing view*, because nurses have a view about many issues affecting health. It is these that need to be clearly articulated by nurses so that a *health view* is given.

Within these new arenas nurses will also need to speak the same language as others, if they are not to be marginalised. Visibility is implicit in nurses having a belief in what they offer, being confident and developing a 'can do' attitude. As Sue Antrobus points out, nurses need to translate their intelligence into a language understood by all those involved in the commissioning process. The nature and value of *caring* need to be expressed and the promotion of services that provide effective, caring, patient-centred interventions needs to be discussed in a language that is understood by others involved in the commissioning process.

Relationships and networks

Effective and successful policy development is dependent on two things: relationships and intelligence gathering. The importance of developing a range of different networks has been emphasised by a number of the contributors. Sandra Rote, for example, in her examination of the nurse role in PCGs, suggests that nurses need to recognise the importance of networking and influencing outside of the board meetings: *nurses may well find that they can achieve more outside of a meeting that during it.*

However, relationships and networks need to move beyond the immediate environs of one's role and job. Nurses have to be seen as effective key facilitators of communication at a local and operational level within the healthcare team. But to exert influence at a policy level, nurses need also to be building relationships, exerting influence and gathering intelligence among legislative, political and academic communities. Moreover, if nurses are going to develop closer links with political, academic and legislative bodies they will need to understand the role and context in which such bodies/communities operate. This means developing a 360-degree outlook in relation to single-issue local issues that effect healthcare delivery. To date, nurses engaged in practice have not necessarily demonstrated strategic skills in this way. The shift required is illustrated in Figure 8.1. Previously, nurses have established professional relationships and networks with professional bodies, doctors and managers. In the future, they need to 'stretch out' further and extend their networks to other academic and legislative bodies.

Implicit in building effective and appropriate networks is the need to understand the cyclical nature of the policy process and to be aware of how to gain access to this. The importance of this understanding has been alluded to by a number of the contributors, but perhaps no more starkly than in the chapter written by Lance Gardener. His very personal story about the development of a nurse-led PCAP pilot in Salford clearly illustrates the importance of understanding how policy and its development is part of a broader legislative and state structure. Lance very quickly learnt that the only way to be effective was to understand the 'big picture' politically and ideologically. That

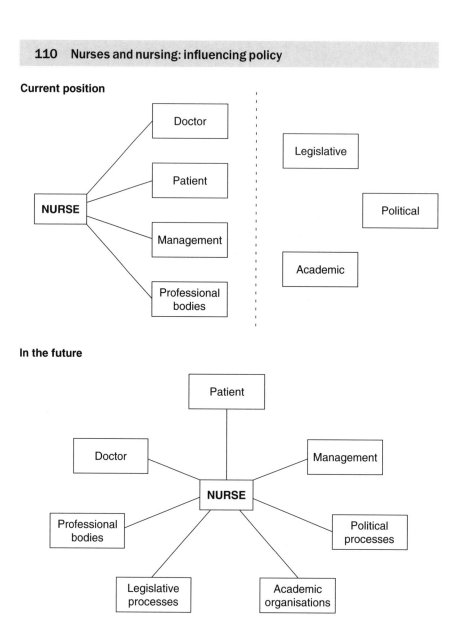

Figure 8.1: Relationships and networks: current position and in the future.

is, to take a whole-systems approach. The current government's preoccupation with 'joined-up thinking' reflects and reinforces the importance of this on a national scale. The increasing importance of a European dimension is not to be forgotten. Europe being part of the whole system is a sentiment reflected in the chapter written by Susan Williams. There is no point revolutionising public health in the UK without reference to public health policy in Europe.

A solution-focused approach

Finally, being positive and seeing not the problems faced by nurses and nursing but rather the challenges with which nurses can engage, will be attractive to others. It is recognised that nurses have been and are marginalised. The challenge is for nurses to shed their victim role and to talk not about the problems but the solutions. Again, Lance has clearly illustrated to us the enormous strides that can be made if problems are posed positively. The example he cites is of a group of nurses involved in PCAP schemes getting together and orchestrating a co-ordinated campaign to inform the nursing media, government ministers and professional bodies about the limitations PCAP nurses faced under the 1992 Prescription by Nurses Act.[1] The solution suggested by the nurses that the Crown review or an amendment to the NHS Act could be used as a vehicle to legitimise prescribing rights for nurses leading a PCAP pilot has received widespread support.

Policy for nursing

The above themes suggest that for nurses to become proficient policy activists, a number of attributes and skills are required. In particular, nurses need to be *strategists*, they need to see possibilities, work within the 'big picture', shape and influence ideas, and seize opportunities. Nurses will need to understand the use of power and politics and be able to work with national and local priorities.

To develop and generate relationships and networks, nurses

should work where there is energy in the system. Nurses will need to take a whole-systems approach, identify connections, work across boundaries, develop groups, create meaning and identity within their networks, and develop an intelligence-gathering process.

Nurses, like all leaders, will need to be courageous, confident and credible. At times, nurses will need to take risks. They will also need to work hard, to know the 'business' they are in and be able to present their ideas clearly to a wide range of bodies.

Finally, nurses who are involved in influencing policy development will need to be reflective. It will be important for them to learn from previous experiences and keep their own knowledge base up to date. As leaders influencing policy, it is also important for nurses to develop others and recognise their own role as role models for others. Nurses involved in influencing policy will therefore need to be learners and developers.

These attributes, when listed together like this, have significant resonance with those attributes found in people with leadership qualities. Ultimately, perhaps this is what we are saying, that if we encourage nurses to become leaders we are also developing their ability to shape policy and influence the political process. Policy will then be formulated *for* nursing as well as just being *of* nursing.

References

1   Department of Health (1992) *Prescription by Nurses Act.* HMSO, London.

Index